F

by **Bob Bent**

illustrated by **Jack Bozzi**

REVISED AND UPDATED

A FIRESIDE BOOK
Published by Simon and Schuster
New York

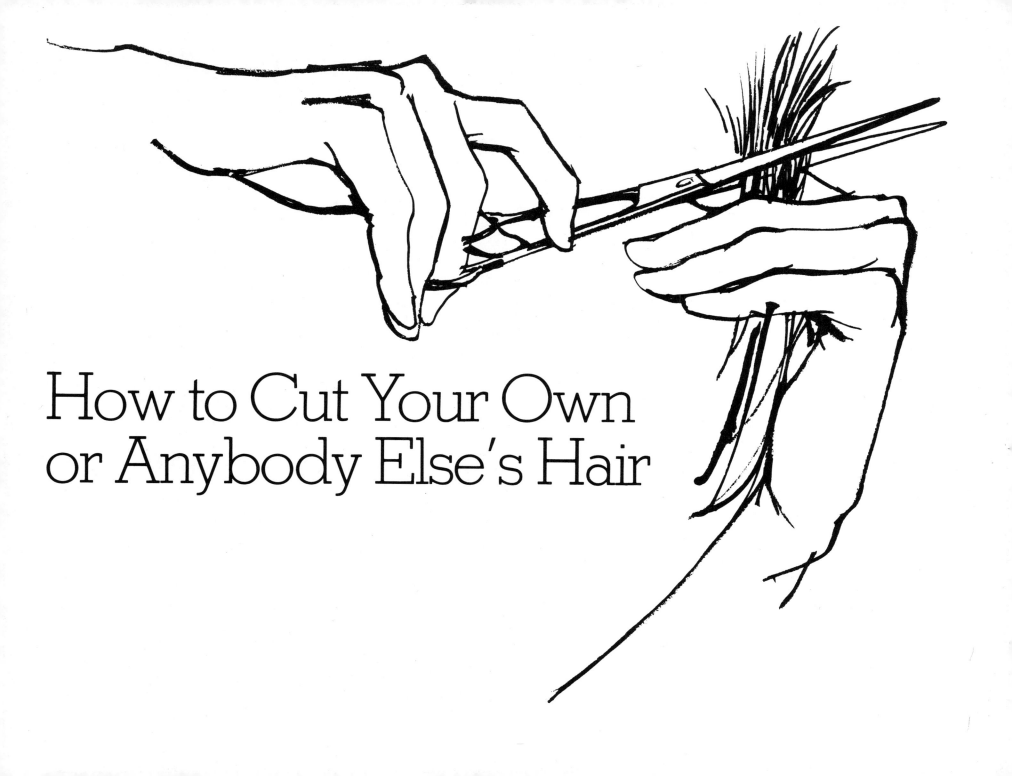
How to Cut Your Own or Anybody Else's Hair

Copyright © 1975, 1983 by Robert Bent and Jack Bozzi
All rights reserved
including the right of reproduction
in whole or in part in any form
Revised Fireside Edition, 1983
Published by Simon & Schuster, Inc.
Simon & Schuster Building
Rockefeller Center
1230 Avenue of the Americas
New York, New York 10020
FIRESIDE and colophon are registered trademarks of Simon & Schuster, Inc.
Manufactured in the United States of America
10 9 8 7
Library of Congress Cataloging in Publication Data
Bent, Bob.
   How to cut your own or anybody else's hair.
   "A Fireside book."
   1. Haircutting. I. Bozzi, Jack. II. Title.
TT970.B46   1983   646.7'24   82-19543
ISBN 0-671-46776-X Pbk.

Contents

Preface to the Revised Edition ... 7
Introduction ... 11

1 What is hair? ... 13

2 What should hair do? ... 17

3 What should you do to your hair? ... 21
    Preparation ... 25

4 The Cuts ... 31
    The Short Cut ... 33
    The Layered Cut ... 54
    The "Punk" Cut ... 71
    The Long Cut ... 77
    The One-Length Cut ... 80

5 How to Cut Children's Hair ... 89
    Short Hair—Straight ... 91
    Short Hair—Curly ... 97
    Long Hair ... 103

6 How to Blow-Dry Your Hair ... 107
    Long Hair Turned Under ... 110
    Long Hair Turned Up (Flip) ... 116
    Short Hair Away from the Face ... 117
    Short Hair Toward the Face ... 122
    Men's Hair ... 127

Preface to Revised Edition

When this book was first published, a great many men and women were wearing their hair in the styles of the late sixties and seventies. Now, perhaps reflecting our busier, more physical lives—we exercise, more, eat better, and work harder—hairstyles are shorter. This new edition will reflect those changes by offering both shorter haircuts and some new advice designed to maintain a haircut so that it looks good and lasts longer.

Even though times have changed, basic haircutting techniques have not. And the tools of the trade remain the same. New scissors have been developed which stay sharper longer and are scientifically designed to last a lifetime, but these are very expensive and are essentially made for the professional haircutter who uses them many hours every day. Home haircutting requires just a few basic tools, all of which are very inexpensive, and in fact, are probably in your home already—so that in many cases there is nothing to buy. Be sure and read the chapter entitled Preparation before you begin, however, just to make sure that you have everything you need. Please read the *entire* book all the way through before you attempt a haircut. Remember, you are learning something new—whether you intend to cut your own or someone else's hair—and it is important to get a *feeling* for the whole process. Reading the entire book will help you to develop this feeling. Then you need practice. Learning to maintain a haircut is a good way to start. Begin by trimming the haircut you already have. It will prepare you for a bigger change.

Learning to maintain your bangs, for instance, very often gives new life to a haircut. You may not always want a complete haircut; yet anyone who wears bangs knows that they are the first part of the cut that begins to annoy, by growing into your eyes and obstructing your vision. Now you can maintain the length of your bangs easily by following the instructions included in this new edition. It is very important to remember always to leave your bangs *longer* than you want them when cutting wet hair. Once your bangs have dried, they will always be shorter, and it is much easier to trim them *dry* if they are still bothering you. Bangs cut too short can be a disaster, and they never seem to grow back fast enough. By taking your time, looking at the illustrations, and cutting a little at a time, such potential disasters can be avoided.

A great many people have used this book to learn to cut their own hair, but many more use it as a manual to cut someone else's hair. I have therefore included in this edition more cuts designed for this second group. Jack Bozzi has refined many of his drawings so that the reader can see the haircutting process close up. He has included the hands of the cutter (working on someone else) so that you can see exactly what it looks like when you are working in front of a mirror. This, I think, is of enormous help to those of you who like to cut other people's hair. These new drawings are clearer and easier to understand—like a lens on a camera which brings the action in for a close-up look. They are also an invaluable aid to those of you who cut your own hair—as you cut in front of a mirror, the new drawings come alive.

Although there are many new drawings of *short* haircuts, long hair has not been neglected. The long cuts remain, and this time I have included a classic one-length above-the-shoulders style which can be worn with or without bangs. Keeping long hair looking healthy and beautiful demands frequent cutting—even if it is only to remove dead ends. I hope that the long haircuts included in these pages will help you to keep your hair looking good and at the same time save you a great deal of money.

I have also included a new section on blow drying for men. It is not at all difficult to master, and should be done very quickly and with a cool, or warm (not hot) dryer. Remember, too much heat burns and dries your hair. Don't overdo it. Blow drying is hardly necessary for the New Wave "punk" haircut also included. It is not a haircut for everyone, but in many cases it can look wonderful. It is definitely one way to have fun with your hair—a real change for those of you who are looking for just that.

We have tried very hard to make these new changes and additions an integral part of the already existing book. Many of the changes are subtle—but clarifying. The most important aspect of this book is simplicity, and this new edition endeavors to keep that intact. Everything has been done in order that you can learn to cut hair better. So read the book and begin cutting. Slowly, please.

Introduction

This book is not intended to replace people who cut hair professionally. After all, *I* cut hair professionally, and I'm very happy at my work. If you've found a hairdresser or barber who cuts your hair well, you'll probably want to stick with him or her. However, if you've always wanted to cut your own hair, or somebody else's, this book will show you how to do it—and how to do it well.

Hair cutting is a skilled craft, and learning to do it well requires good instructions. I've planned this book so that the text and illustrations offer just that—step-by-step instructions that show you exactly how to proceed with assurance. I've included basic hairstyles for men and women and a special chapter on haircuts for children.

A good haircut is vitally important to overall good looks, as anybody who has ever had a bad haircut knows. Finding a cut that complements your features and your hair is an individual matter. It depends on a certain willingness to experiment. Don't make too drastic a change, but do be willing to consider a new look. You cannot change the color of your eyes or the shape of your face, but you can change your hair. You can cut it many different ways and choosing the right length and style is up to you. No matter what kind of hair you have, you should be able to find a cut that works for you among the basic cuts we offer. Obviously not every style works well with every kind of hair, for example: very fine, thin hair does not usually look good in a layered cut. I offer some general rules about choosing the right haircut in Chapter 2.

Before you choose the cut you want and start cutting, I suggest that you read the book all the way through, including chapters that don't seem to apply to you. Even if you plan to cut an adult's hair, you can get good ideas from the children's chapter. So read it all first and then choose the chapter that shows the haircut you want. Then follow the directions carefully, take your time, and you should be assured of achieving the look you want. It's exciting to learn to do something well, and you may even discover that you have a real talent for haircutting.

1
What is hair?

Hair is a threadlike outgrowth of minute depressed pockets in the scalp known as "follicles." The shape of the follicle determines the type of hair you have.

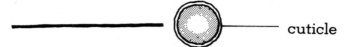

A round follicle produces straight hair

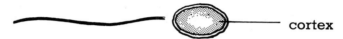

An oval follicle produces curly hair

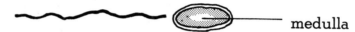

A flat follicle produces kinky hair

So the kind of hair you have is determined before it grows out of the scalp. Of course, you can change it if you wish (through permanent waving or straightening), but either of these can be a pretty damaging procedure. As your hair grows in, the new growth will be in its natural state and you'll be involved in a continual cycle of curling or straightening it. Naturally, this is also true if you use permanent hair color. I'm not saying that you should not do any of these things. On the contrary, sometimes a slight permanent wave, color change or straightening can be beautiful. But it should be slight, so that when the hair grows in it will blend with the changed part.

Generally, however, I feel that hair should be left alone to grow as it will. Healthy, natural hair looks best—if it's cut properly.

Looking at a single strand of hair under a microscope reveals this:

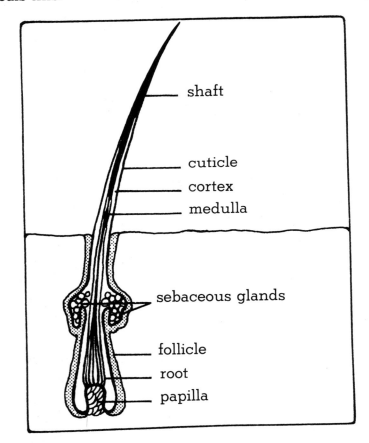

The color of your hair is determined by pigments in the middle layer—the cortex. These pigments sometimes darken with age, and can also get lighter when exposed to the sun. Generally, however, the pigment remains pretty much the same for most of one's life, until it gradually fades and produces gray hair. You can change this by adding color to your hair. If you do decide to color your hair, it should be done gently, using a solution that does not permanently color the hair, but rather one which gradually washes out and needs to be redone. These "color baths" (products with no peroxide) are the best way to cover gray. My suggestion is to stay as close to your natural color as possible and to use the gentlest solution.

Hair grows out approximately 1/2 inch a month. This varies a little with the seasons—slower in winter and faster in summer. If you have short hair and decide to let it grow out into a longer style, regular cutting and trimming about six or eight weeks apart can help to keep your hair healthy and attractive while it's growing. That way you'll look good while you wait and prevent irreparable damage to your hair. Don't use products to stimulate growth. They don't work. Just be patient and before long you will have the length you want.

Also, hair is constantly replacing itself, so don't worry if some hair comes out when you are combing or brushing. You can use your own judgment as to whether or not you feel that the hair coming out is really excessive. If you notice an abnormal amount, go to a scalp specialist and let him decide.

Remember: with the proper diet and care, your hair can be what it should be—healthy and beautiful. Forget the gimmicks, and let your hair breathe and grow freely. Then cut it right.

2
What should hair do?

Hair should be free. It should move freely, blow in the wind, and still look great. And there is only one way to have this kind of hair—with a good haircut. A haircut that complements you and your hair gives you a sense of freedom and natural good looks.

When choosing the length and cut you want, you should think of all the times you've looked your best and you'll be able to choose what really works well for you. Some people seem to be able to wear almost any hairstyle, but they are exceptions. People who are incredibly beautiful can wear their hair down to their knees or an inch long all over their heads and still look great. But even the beautiful benefit from a good cut—they look even better.

As you will see, hair is cut the same way for men and women. Generally speaking, men can go shorter than women without looking shorn. Also, many men do not know how to handle the longer haircuts and their hair can get to look unkempt. But hair length is a very personal choice, and you'll know what is right for you.

Many people decide to cut their hair when they're feeling dissatisfied with themselves or their lives. That's OK because a new haircut can really lift your spirits; but I'd like to add a word of warning here. Don't cut your hair when you're angry—disaster is certain. Put on some music you love and sit down with this book and go through it until you're relaxed and can choose wisely. Sit back and really think about your hair and you'll come to a well thought-out decision that you'll be happy about later.

I'll offer a few general rules that do not apply in all cases, but do in most:

1. Heavy people usually do not look good in very short hair. It tends to make them look bottom-heavy and pointed on top.
2. People with fine, straight hair should almost never layer their hair. A one-length blunt cut is best unless it is cut very short.
3. Very curly, almost kinky hair should definitely be layered, otherwise it will fly out and give too much width.
4. Thin people often seem to disappear when they have very short hair, unless they are very tall—in which case it can be great.
5. Very thin hair looks best short—it makes it look thicker.
6. Very thick hair is probably the biggest problem to cut. It can look fine any way, but deciding how it should be cut can be difficult. Experimenting with different styles seems to be the only answer —it will grow.

How you wear your hair is probably the first thing people notice about you—as well as what you yourself notice first when you look in a mirror. The mirror doesn't lie. Keep in mind that your hair should complement your face and body. Don't be intimidated by your hair—afraid of cutting it because you are not sure what it will do when cut. Try a few styles and you're bound to find one that suits you. There is no reason for fear. Let your mind and your mirror make the decision—you'll never find what's right for you without trying. A word of warning: Don't cut very long hair very short all at once—do it gradually.

A haircut should not be a shock, it should be a beautiful surprise.

3
What should you do to your hair?

Love your hair. Shampoo it often. Brush it. Treat it like a friend. Hair that is well cared for looks it.

There are several important steps in caring for your hair and the first is to cut it fairly often—once every six or eight weeks. If you let your hair grow for longer periods, the ends will split and your hair will tangle. That's when the damage starts. When you comb or brush hair that has split ends, it will break off, leaving short pieces that fly away from your head. So, it's very important to cut your hair often, even if you just cut off the very ends.

To brush or not to brush seems to be the great debate currently, and it shouldn't be. It's clear to me that the right kind of brushing is good for hair. I suggest brushing your hair for a few minutes every day. It should be brushed from the scalp all the way to the ends, in order to distribute the natural oils all along the hair shaft. Use a natural bristle brush and try to get into the habit of brushing before going to bed. Also, keep your brush clean by washing it in warm water with a little shampoo—then let it dry by itself.

After shampooing, comb your hair with the wide teeth of the comb first. Never pull out the snarls. Work them out gently until the fine teeth go through your hair easily.

If you wash your hair often (every day or two) don't blow-dry every time. Heat hurts. Use your own good judgment and when you do blow-dry your hair, don't use a hot dryer—use a warm one. Overexposure to heat can make the hair dry and brittle. There's a special chapter on how to blow-dry your hair at the end of the book.

Following a few simple rules should leave your hair healthy and lustrous.

I don't think using sticky cream rinses is good for the hair. They leave a residue on the hair shaft that attracts dirt and grime. When you do condition your hair, use a first-rate conditioner and set aside some time to let it work. Use the best products available and indulge yourself and your hair. Once a week is more than enough—never more than that, and for most people twice a month is sufficient.

Use a conditioner that stays on your head for about half an hour (hot olive oil is great), and wrap your head in hot towels to let the conditioner really penetrate the hair shaft. Use just a small amount of oil. In between treatments you can use a balsam product—on fine hair use about half the recommended amount—but not every time you shampoo.

The most important thing I can tell you is to be aware of your hair. Don't overdo anything. If you treat your hair with the greatest of care, you can't go wrong.

Preparation

A good haircut always begins with a good shampoo. *Never* cut your own hair or anyone else's when it's dry. Find a good natural shampoo with as little detergent as possible—preferably none. Castile shampoos are natural and gentle. If you shampoo your hair almost every day, give yourself one good soaping and rinse thoroughly. If you only have to wash your hair twice a week, give yourself two soapings, the first to remove the surface dirt, and the second to massage and clean the scalp. (Washing your hair once a week is simply not enough. It should be done at least twice to keep your hair clean and shiny.) After the shampoo, comb your hair gently with a wide-tooth comb. Do not pull it hard. Take your time and slowly comb through small sections of hair until you can freely comb all the hair straight back away from your face. After you've combed out your clean wet hair you are ready to cut. Since you want to be free to move around, don't wear a bathrobe or shirt.

Equipment you'll need
1. Two mirrors—one to face and the other positioned so that you can see the back of your head. Obviously, you don't need these if you're cutting somebody else's hair, but it's a good idea for the person who's getting the haircut to face a mirror so he or she can see what's happening and comment on what they'd like.
2. A standard barber's comb. This is a narrow comb that has both fine and wide teeth. It's about 8 inches long.
3. A good pair of cutting shears. Don't spare the ex-

pense on the scissors. This is your most important piece of equipment. Buy a good sharp pair, as small as possible, about 5 or 6 inches.
4. A couple of large hair clips, about 3 or 4 inches long. These are used to hold up the hair before you cut it. (If you want, you can use rubber bands to hold hair, but I suggest clips.)

If you're cutting your own hair, here are some rules to follow:
1. All cuts should be made while you're facing the mirror.
2. Always cut with the same hand that holds the comb. In other words, when you are working, put down the comb and pick up the scissors with the *same* hand.
3. Always cut off the hair in front of your fingers, never behind, so that the hair falls away from you as you cut.

Now you're ready to cut. Put the book down on a counter or table in front of you—relax—and begin.

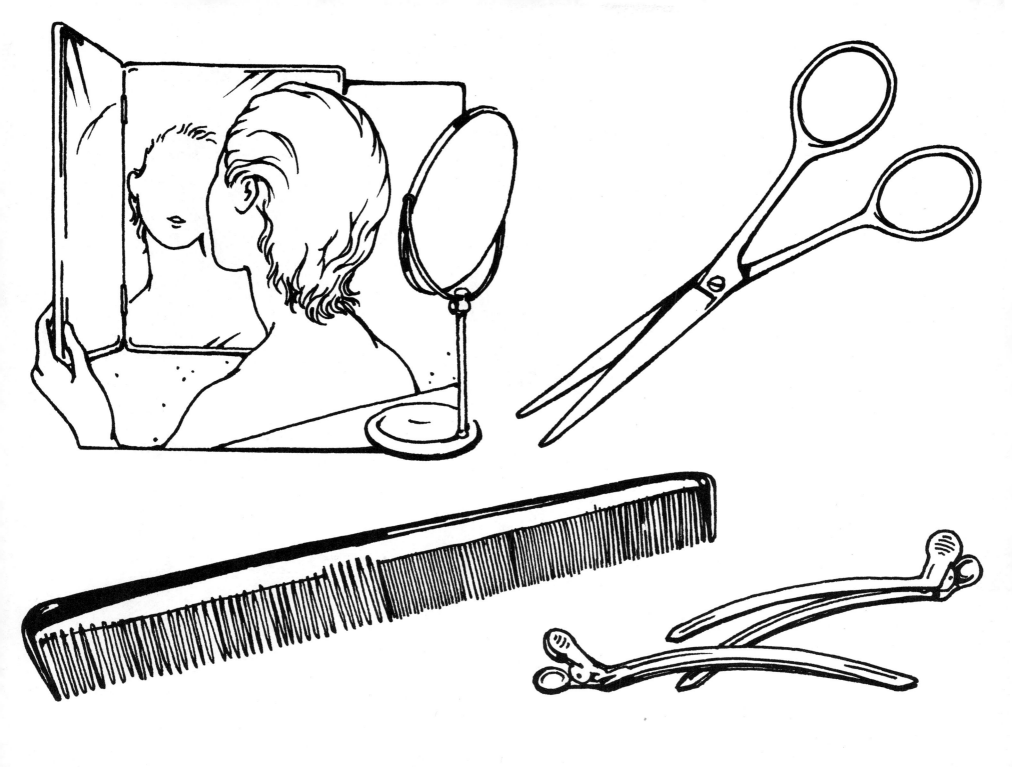

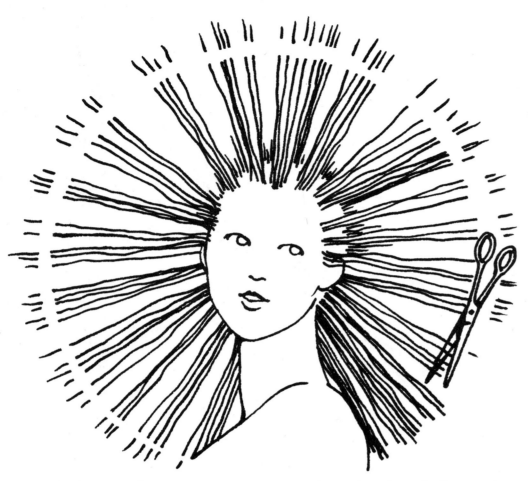

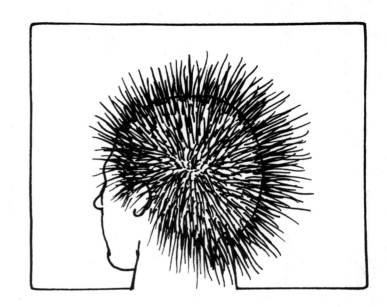

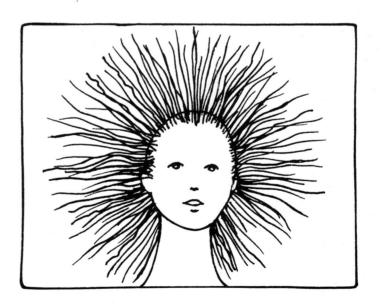

Before you begin cutting, you must have an idea of what it is you want to accomplish. For our first two cuts, the Short Cut and the Layered Cut, we use what we call the Electrified Image. This is quite simply a view of yourself with all your hair standing on end—straight out from your scalp. Keep this image in mind if you are using either of these cuts—it will clarify each succeeding step for you.

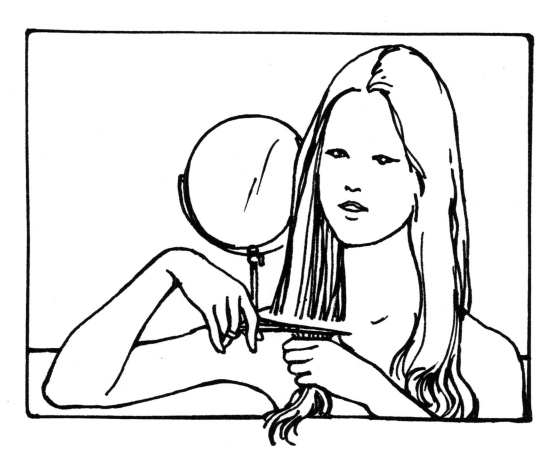

If your hair is very long (below your shoulders), and you plan to give yourself the Layered Cut or the Short Cut, then first part your wet hair in the middle and cut it slightly above your shoulders to avoid complications.

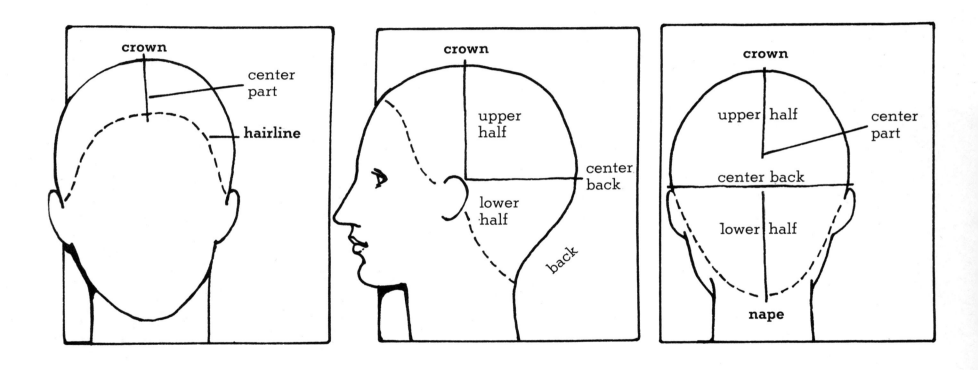

Use this chart to guide you when we refer to these specific parts in the following chapters.

4
The Cuts

The Short Cut

how to cut your own

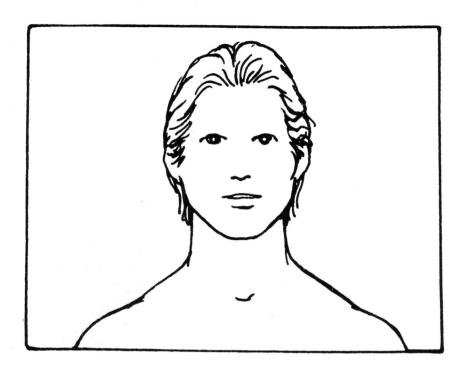

Step 1 Comb wet clean hair straight back away from your face.

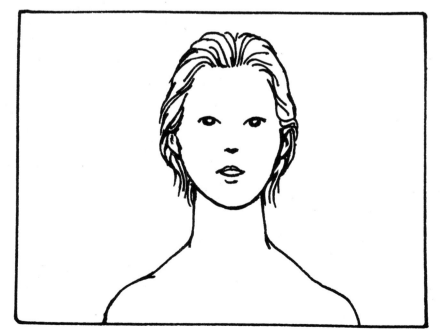

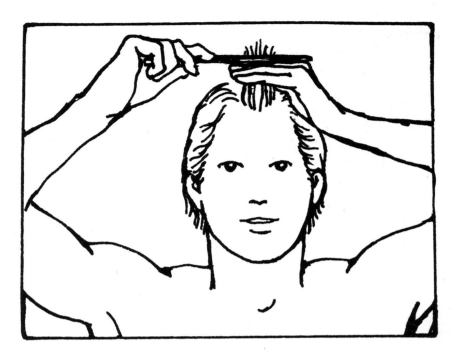

Step 2 Put the comb in the center of your head and pull a small portion of hair straight up, following with your fingers.

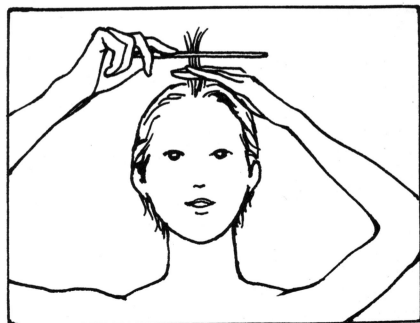

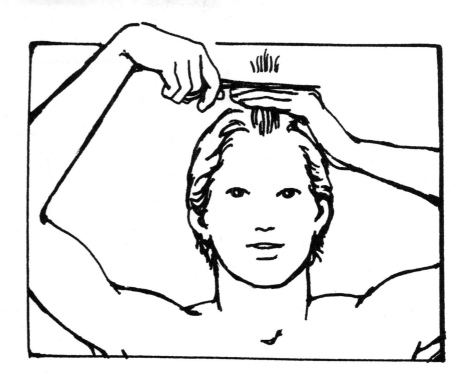

Step 3 Put down the comb while holding the hair up and cut straight across to desired length.

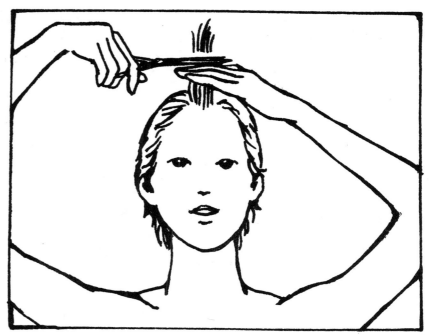

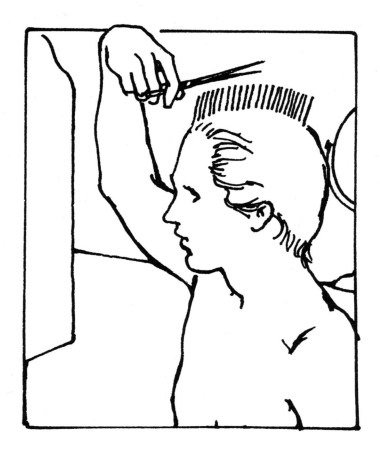

Step 4 Continue this process straight back toward the crown of your head, using what you have just cut as a guide, and cut the entire top of your head the same length, conforming to the contour of your head.

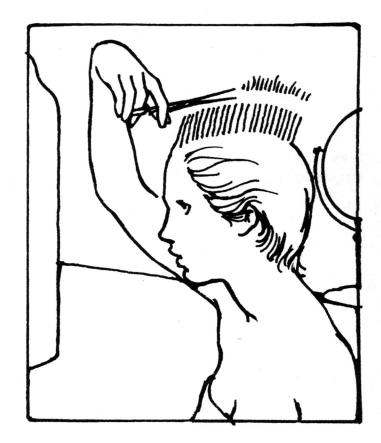

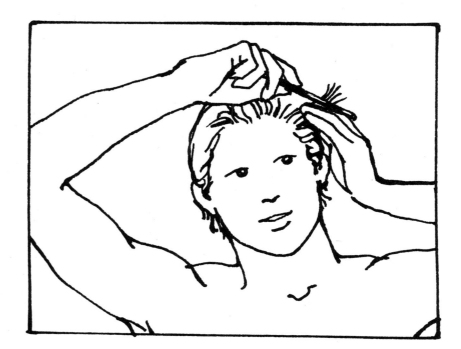

Step 5 Holding the comb at an angle conforming to the angle of the side of your head, pull a small portion of hair straight out of the left side of your head, following with your fingers.

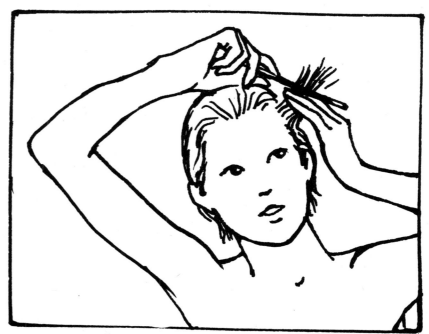

Step 6 Cut the hair, at an angle, the same length as the top.

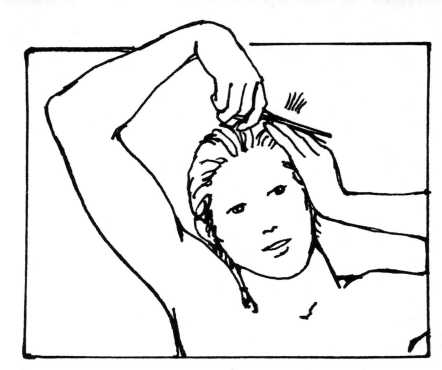
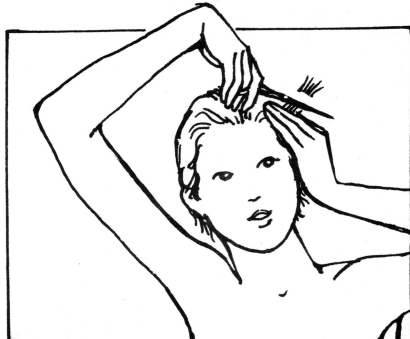

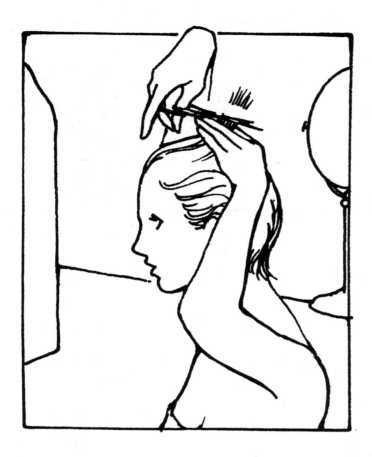

Step 7 Continue combing, pulling out, and cutting the hair the same length all the way along the upper half of your head until you reach the center of the back of your head.

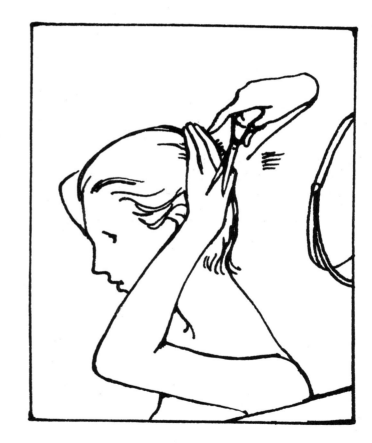

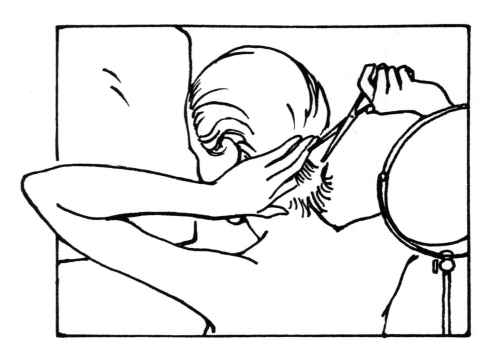

Step 8 Continue this process on the lower part of your head, cutting the hair all the same length until you reach the center of the back of your head.

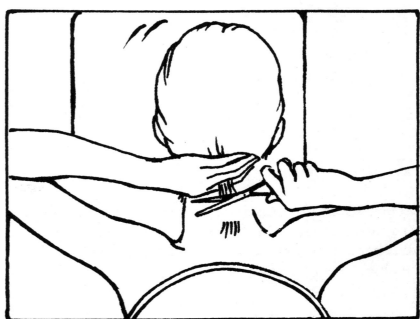

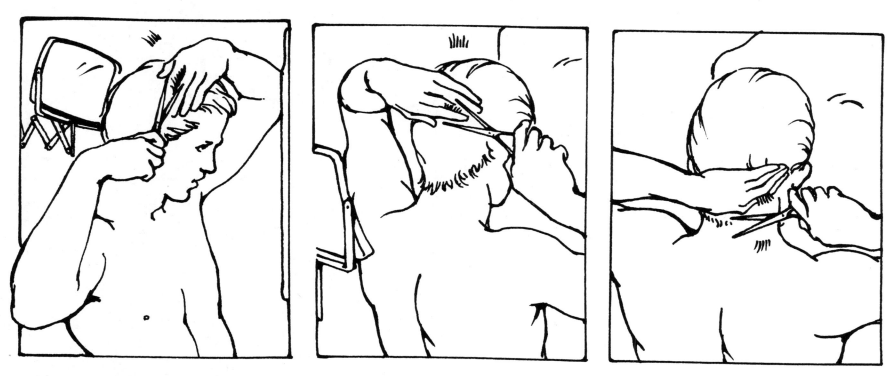

Step 9 When you have finished one side, do the other side exactly the same way—cutting both the upper and lower parts of your hair the same length all the way around to the center of the back. You are forming a circle with all the hair cut the same length.

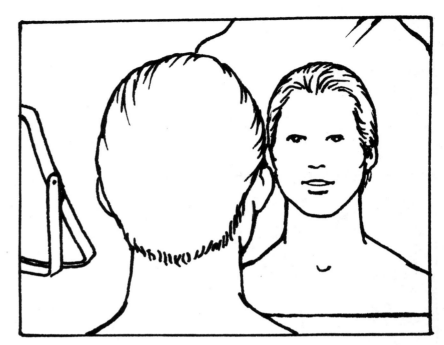

Step 10 Having cut all the hair the same length at this point, comb your hair straight back, and using two mirrors, cut the very bottom as straight across or design the edges as uneven as you wish.

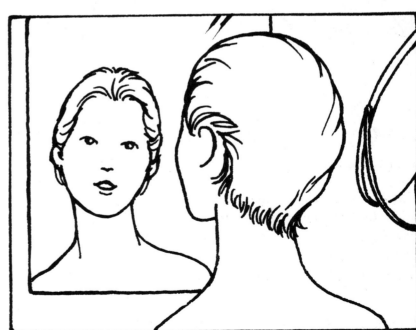

(for men only)
sideburns

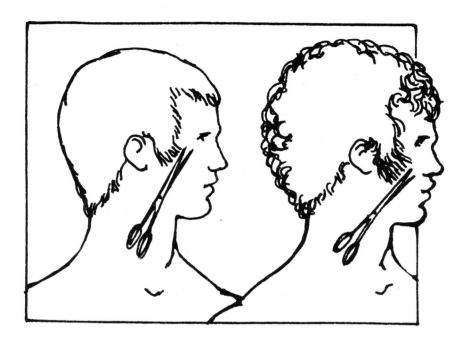

Step 11 Comb the entire sideburn forward and cut off all the ragged edges. Then comb the sideburn straight back and cut it as you like. Trim to your taste around the ears.

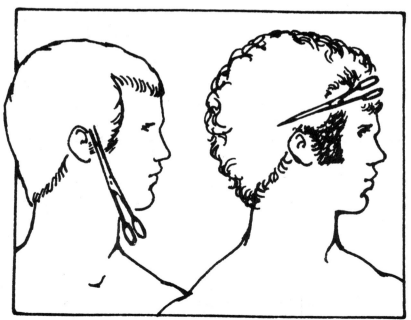

How to Cut Somebody Else's Hair *Very* Short

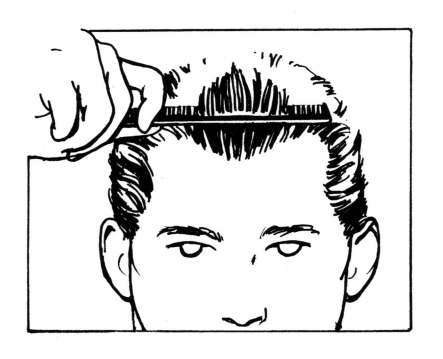 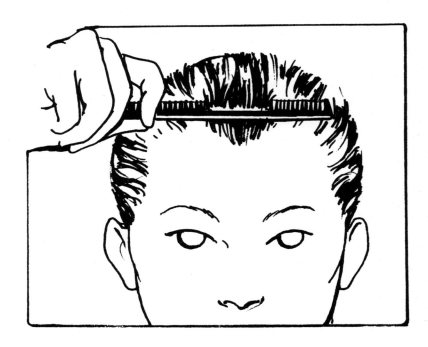

Step 1 Comb wet clean hair straight back away from the face.

Close-Up Version

Step 2 Put the comb in the center of the head and pull a small portion of hair straight up, following with your fingers. Cut just slightly above the width of your fingers.

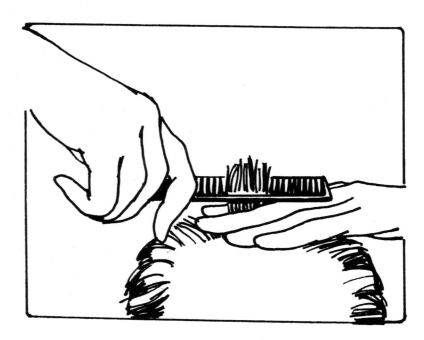

Step 3 Put down the comb (or hold it with the same hand that's holding the hair) and cut the hair straight across to desired length.

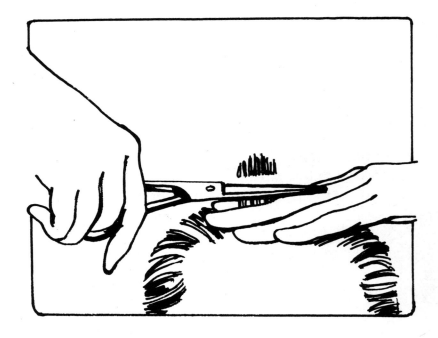

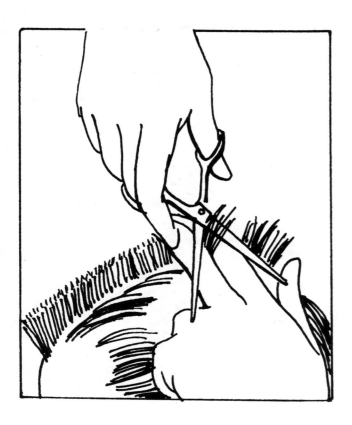 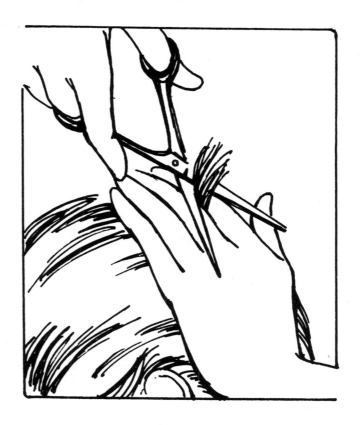

Step 4 Continue this process straight back toward the crown of the head, using what you have just cut as a guide, and cut the entire top of the head the same length, conforming to the contour of the head.

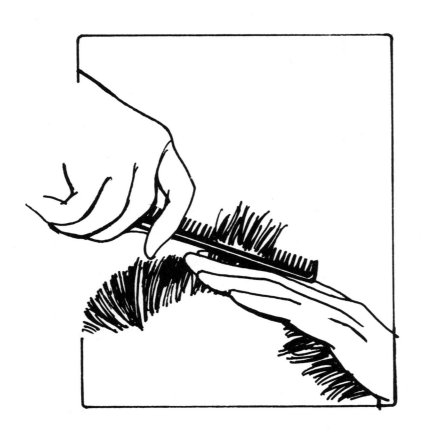 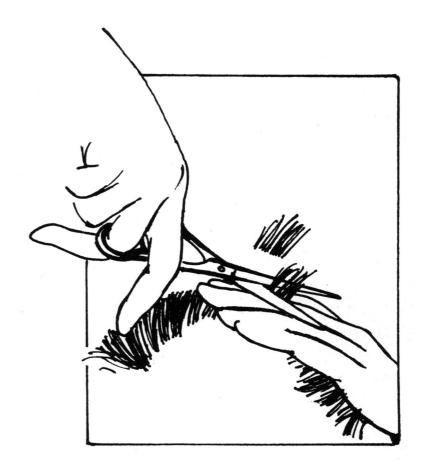

Step 5 Holding the comb on an angle conforming to the angle of the side of the head, pull a small portion of hair straight out of the left side of the head, following with your fingers.

Step 6 Cut the hair, at an angle, the same length as the top.

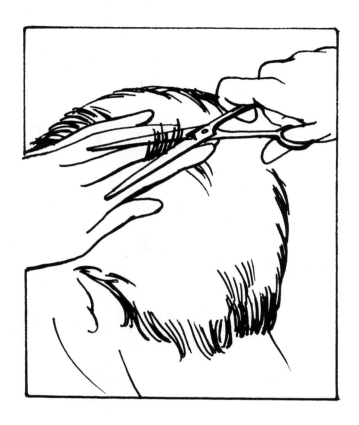

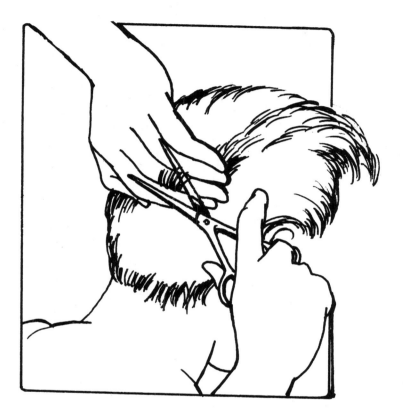

Step 7 Continue combing, pulling out, and cutting the hair the same length all the way along the upper half of the head until you reach the center of the back of the head.

Step 8 Continue this process on the lower half of the head, cutting the hair all the same length until you reach the center of the back of the head.

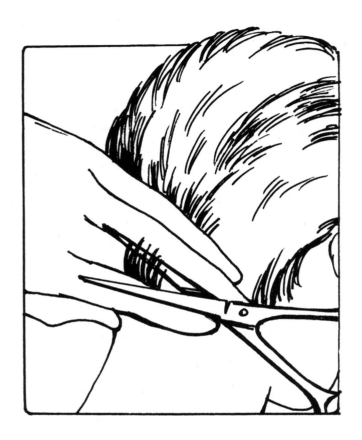

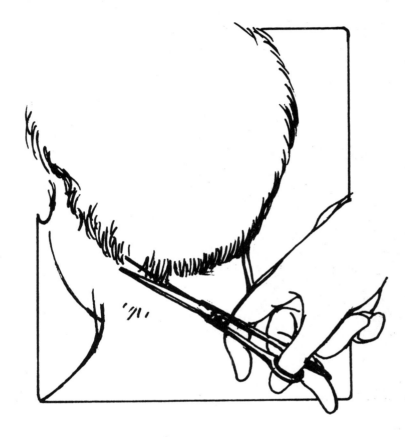

Step 9 When you have finished one side, do the other side exactly the same way—cutting both the upper and lower parts of the hair the same length all the way around to the center of the back. You are forming a circle with all the hair cut the same length.

Step 10 Having cut all the hair the same length, at this point, comb the hair straight back, and cut the very bottom as straight across or design the edges as uneven as you wish.

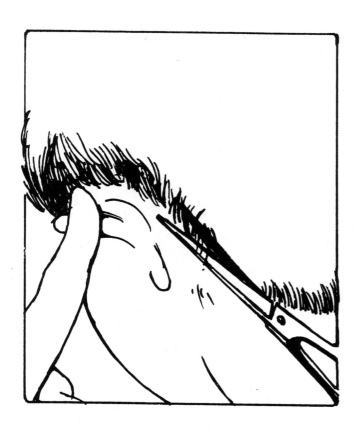 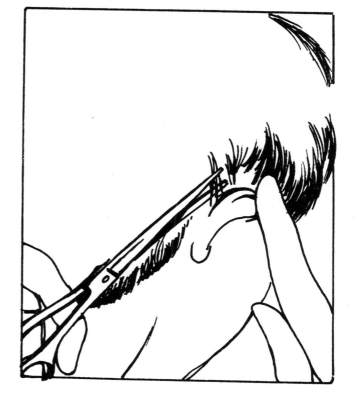

Step 11 When you have finished cutting all around the head, comb hair straight down over ears. Cut around left ear *back* to *front*, if you are right-handed, reverse if lefty. Then do right ear front to back. Be careful—go very *slowly*—cutting a little at a time.

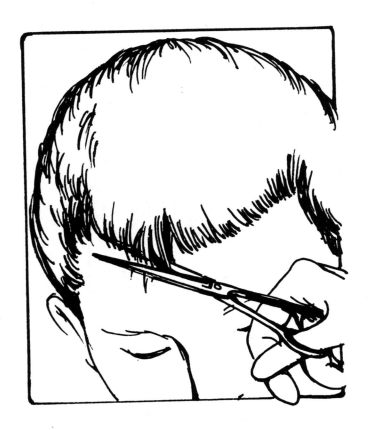

Step 12 Comb the hair straight down in front and cut bang as even or uneven as you wish.

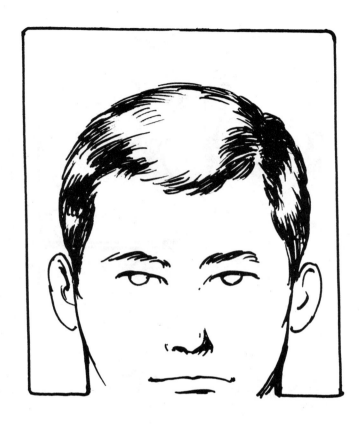 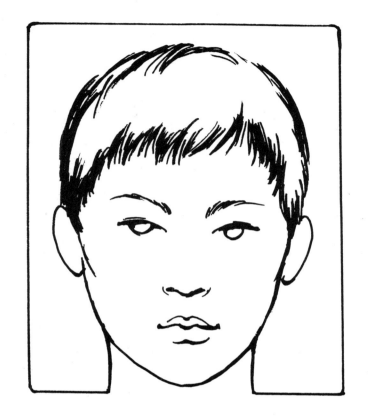

The finished haircut can be worn with or without a part.

The Layered Cut

Step 1 Comb wet clean hair straight back away from your face and part in the middle from your hairline to the nape of your neck.

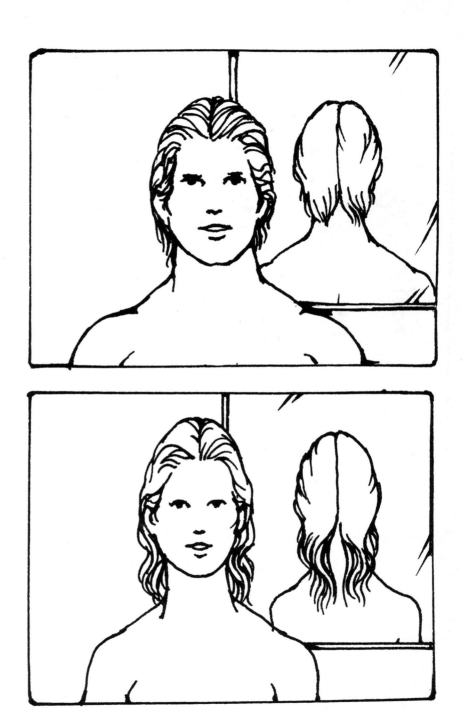

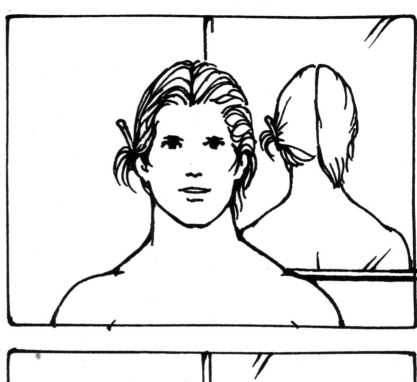

Step 2 Take the right half of your hair and get it out of the way with a clip or rubber band. You will be working with only the left side of your hair for now.

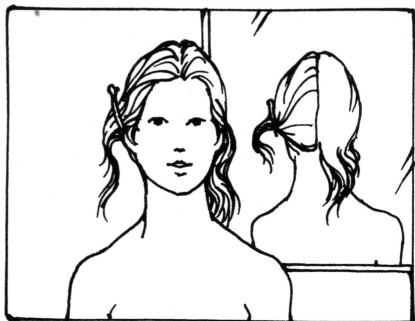

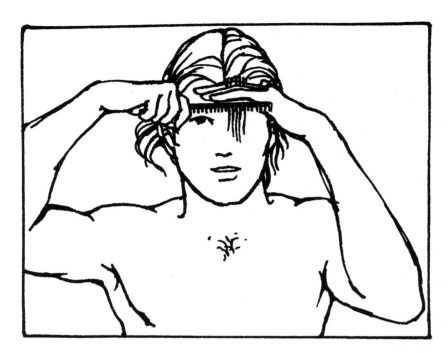

Step 3 With the comb, go 1 inch in from the hairline on the free side (the left) and pull the hair straight forward.

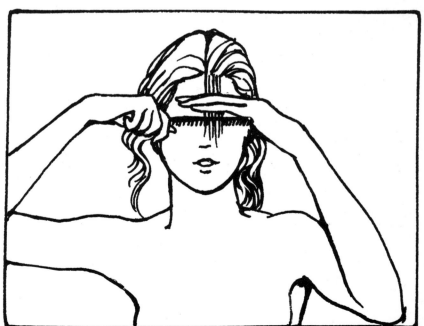

Step 4 Put down the comb while holding the hair you have just pulled out taut with the other hand. Cut off whatever you have decided on, in **front** of your fingers.

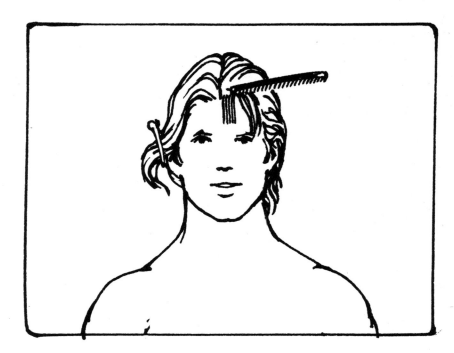

Step 5 Take the comb and make another 1-inch parting (now about 2 inches from the hairline), down toward the ear, and pull forward for the second cut.

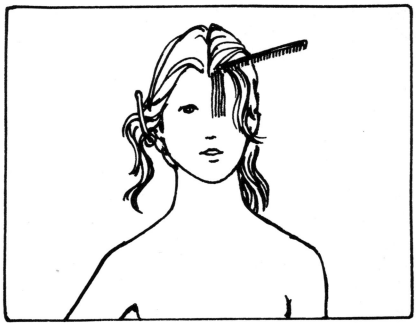

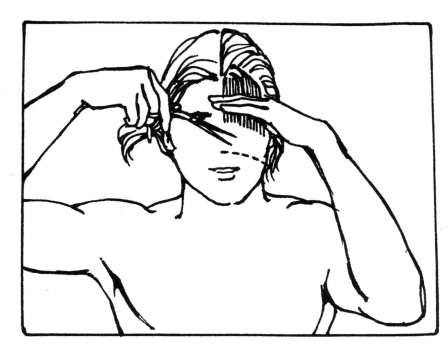

Step 6 Using your first cut as a guide, follow the contour of your head and cut in a semicircle toward the ear.

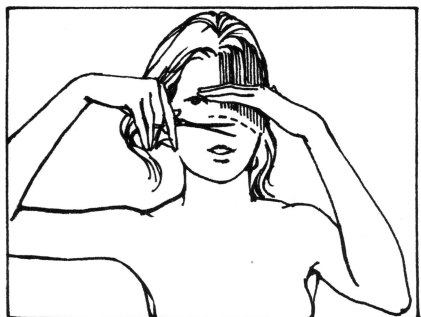

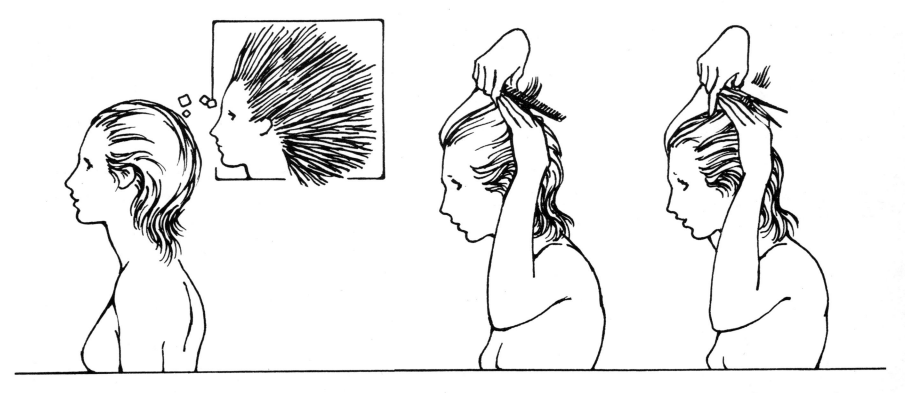

Step 7 Comb the free side straight back and stop. At this point you must imagine your hair in the Electrified Image.

You will begin combing and cutting, conforming to the contour of your head, using the first two cuts as your guide. You will do this until you reach the back center part. Work on the upper half of your hair first.

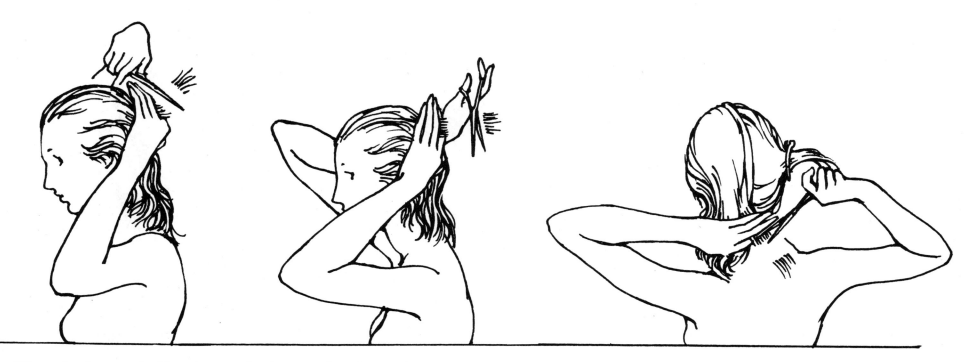

Then the bottom half—cutting the hair to the shape of your fingers, which in turn reflect the shape of your head.

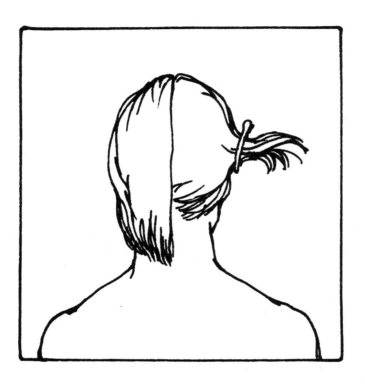 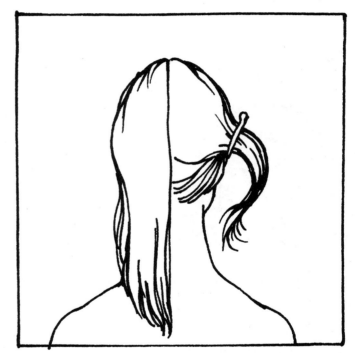

When you reach this point, one whole half of your hair should be cut about the length you want. Don't worry about the very bottom, we will get to that in the final step.

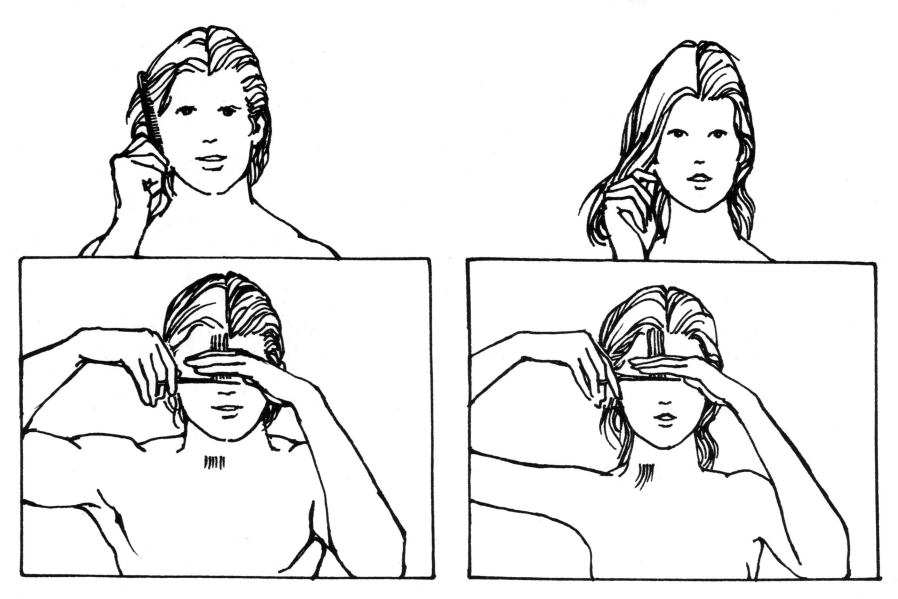

Step 8 Now take down the other side of your hair (the right) and proceed to cut in exactly the same way as you did the left, following each step as we have outlined in the preceding pages.

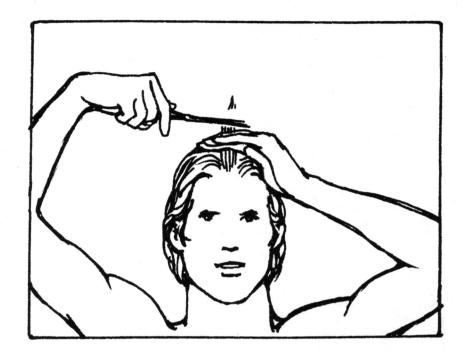

Step 9 When both sides are cut, comb all the hair straight back away from your face. With the comb, pick up the front piece of hair and cut off the edges in a straight line.

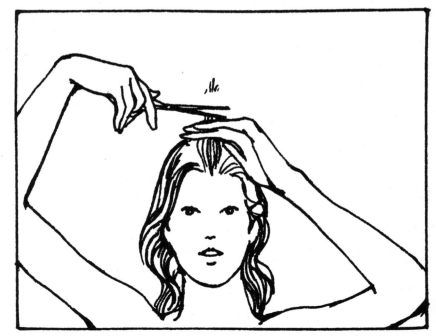

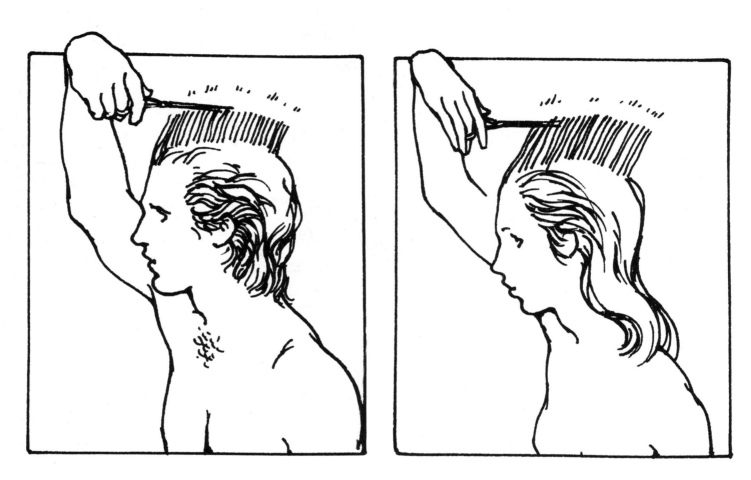

Step 10 Continue back toward the back of your head, using what you have just cut as a guide, and cut the entire top of your head the same length, conforming to the contour of your head.

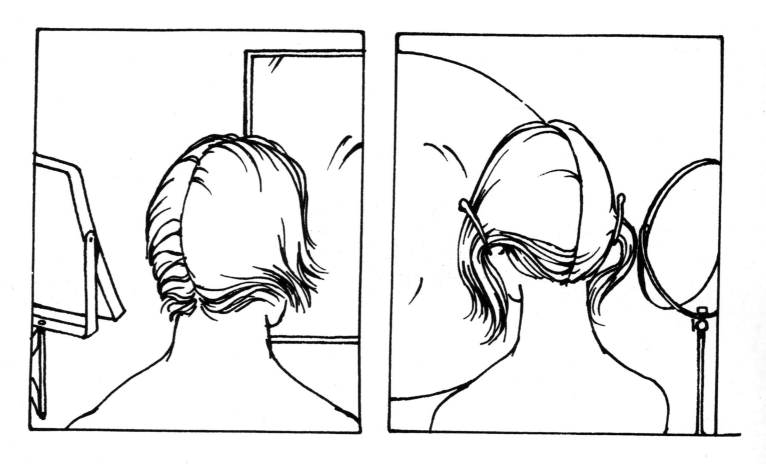

Step 11 Looking in two mirrors, so that you can see the very back of your head, part the hair down the center of the back.

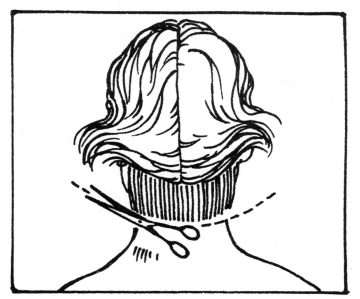
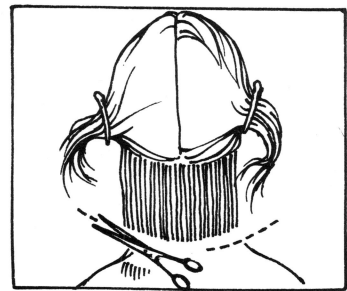

Step 12 With the comb, go 1 inch up from your back hairline, and make a parting from ear to ear. Bring the hair straight down and cut it in an oval shape or straight across as you choose. (We will use the oval shape.)

If the very bottom of your hair is still too long—and you have trouble cutting it looking in the reflection in the rear mirror—pull it forward over your shoulder and cut it in an oval.

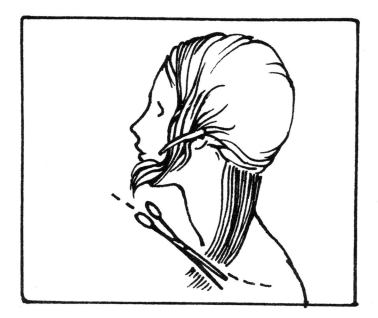

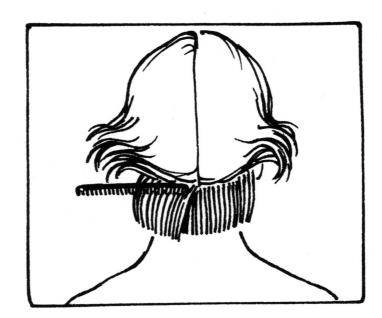

Step 13 Take another 1-inch parting, comb it straight down, and following what you have just cut, cut this new section of hair about 1/4 inch **longer** than the hair underneath (which you have just cut).

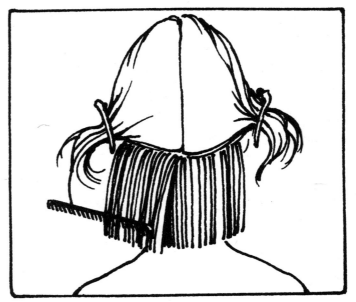

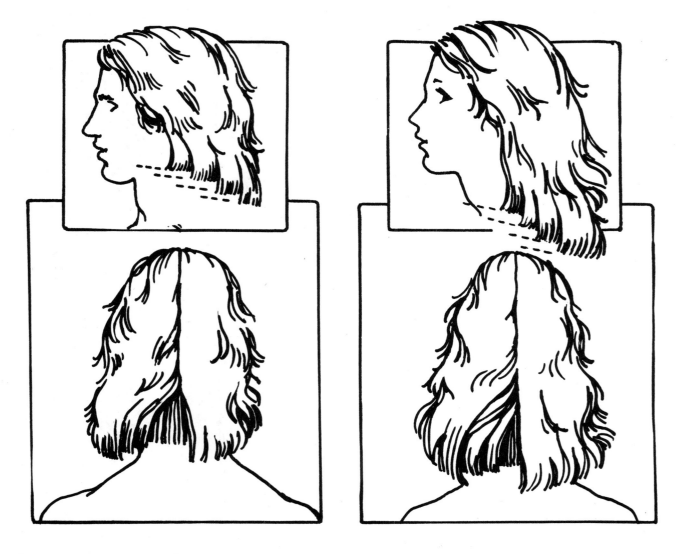

Step 14 Repeat this in 1-inch partings until you can comb all the hair down and there are no ragged edges. Leave each new parting 1/4 inch longer.

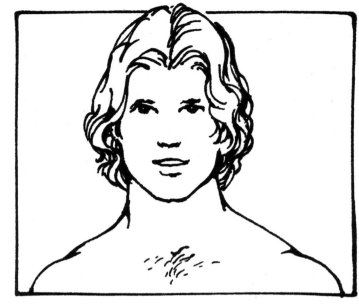

When you are finished, your hair should look like this when mostly dry.

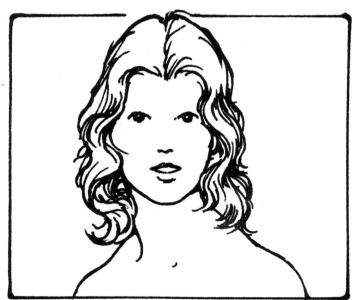

The "Punk" Cut

NOTE: This cut is for men or women. We are going to cut the top short and leave length on the bottom.

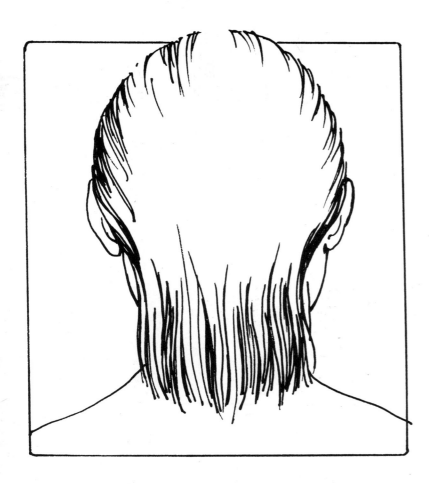

Step 1 Comb wet clean hair back away from the face. We will begin at the back.

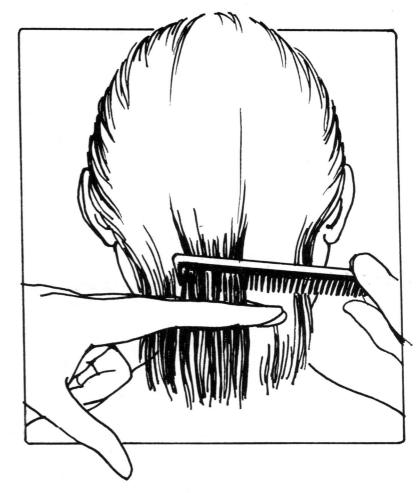

Step 2 Comb through and hold with two fingers at the center of the back of the head—below the hairline, about three quarters of the way down the neck.

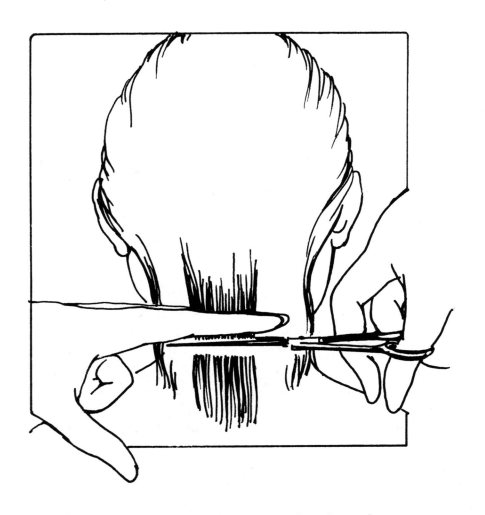

Step 3 Put down the comb and pick up the scissors with your cutting hand. Cut straight across. Under your fingers.

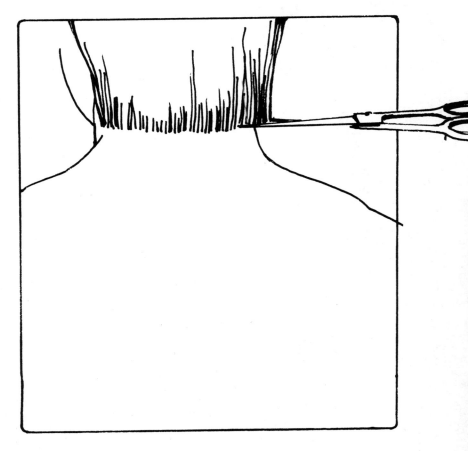

Step 4 Do the same all across the back of the head—both sides of the center you have just cut.

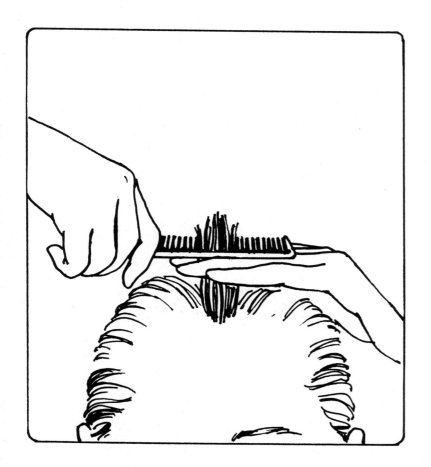

Step 5 Now go to the front hairline. Put the comb in the center of the head and pull a small portion of hair straight up, following with your fingers.

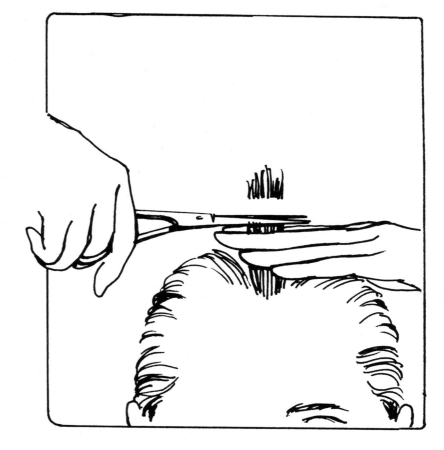

Step 6 Put down the comb and cut the hair straight across to desired length (about 1½ inches from scalp).

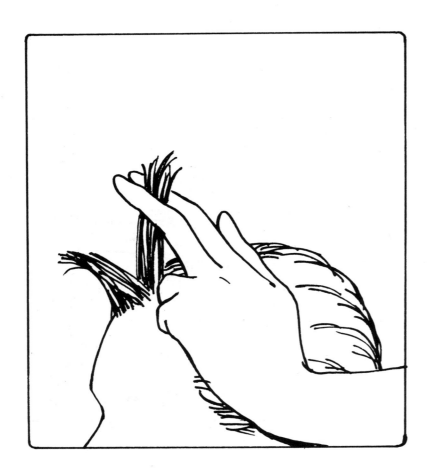 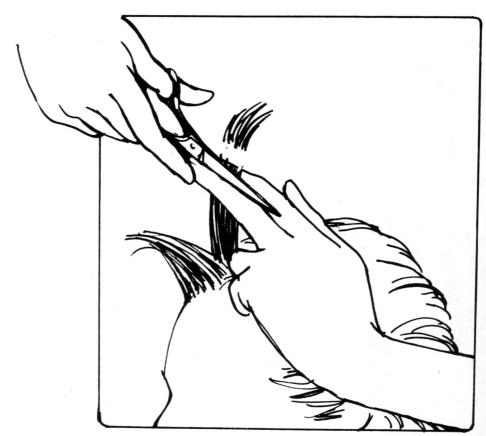

Step 7 Pick up small sections of hair behind the front hair you have just cut. Use your comb and fingers to hold the hair up.

Step 8 Pick up the scissors with your cutting hand and cut this small tuft of hair you are holding. Cut *above* your fingers.

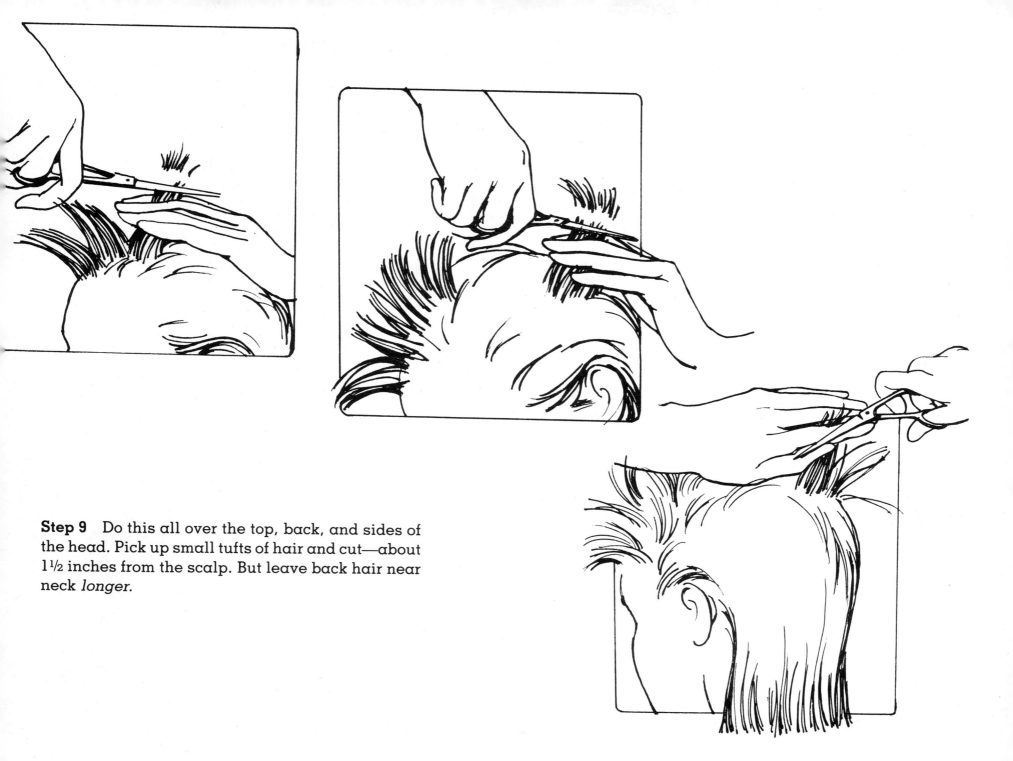

Step 9 Do this all over the top, back, and sides of the head. Pick up small tufts of hair and cut—about 1½ inches from the scalp. But leave back hair near neck *longer*.

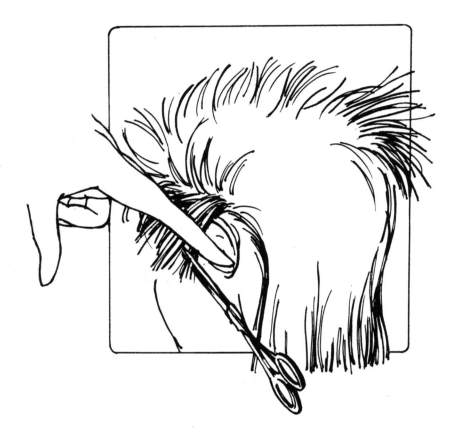

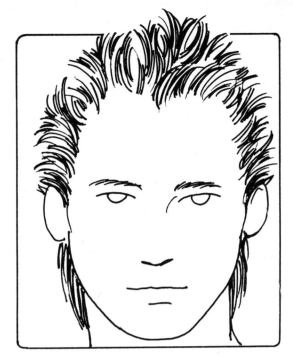

Finished Haircut.

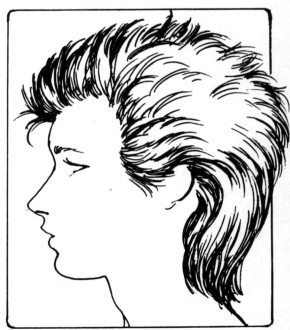

Step 10 When you have finished doing this all over the head, comb hair down on sides and cut around ear as you choose.

The Long Cut

This section will be very brief since it is for people who only want to trim their hair, while leaving it quite long.

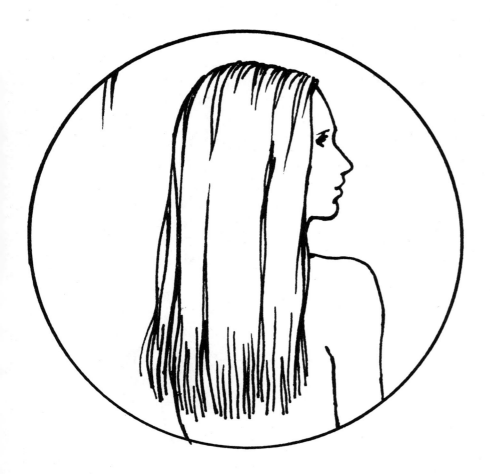

Your idea or image of your hair is very different for our next two sections—the Long Cut and the One-Length Cut.

You should imagine your hair hanging straight down, as if pulled taut by unusually strong gravity.

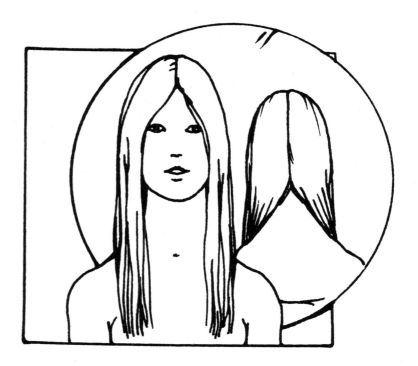

Step 1 Comb wet clean hair straight down, parted in the center from the hairline to the nape of the neck.

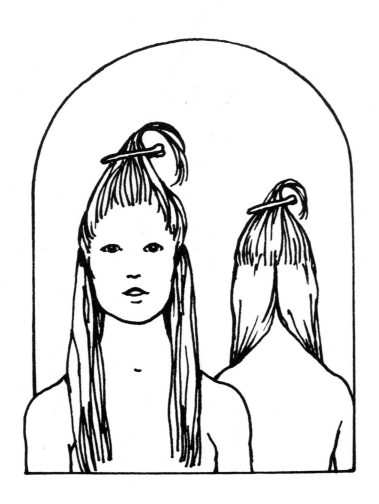

Step 2 Divide your hair into two halves —upper and lower—getting the upper portion out of the way with a clip or rubber band.

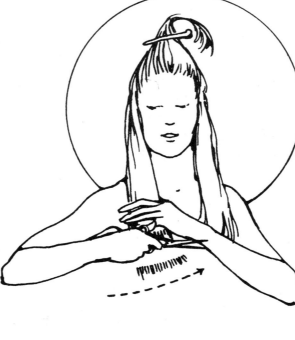

Step 3 Pull each side forward, including the back all the way to the center part, and cut off as much as you want. Cut it in a slight angle toward the back for the oval shape.

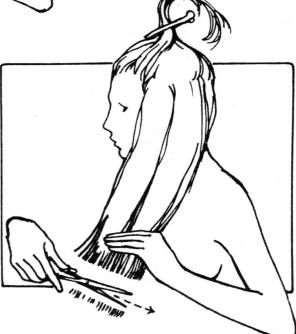

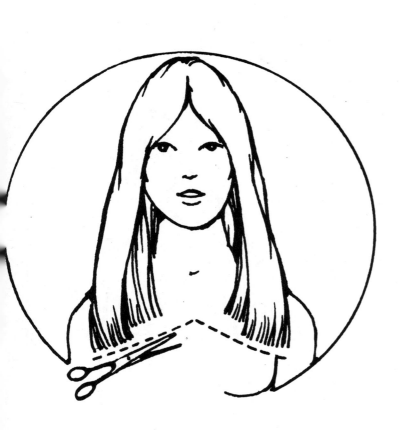

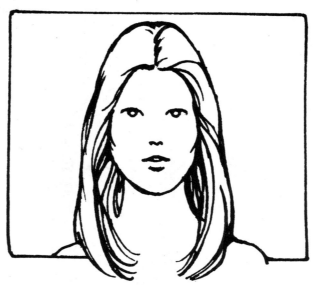

When you are finished, your hair should look like this.

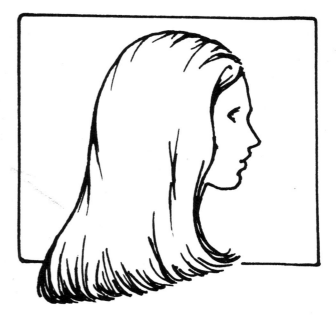

Step 4 Take down the top half and do the same. Pull all the hair forward over the hair you have just cut and cut it about 1/2 inch longer, using what you have already cut as a guide. This will allow your hair, when dry, to turn under slightly naturally.

79

The One-Length Cut (with Bangs)

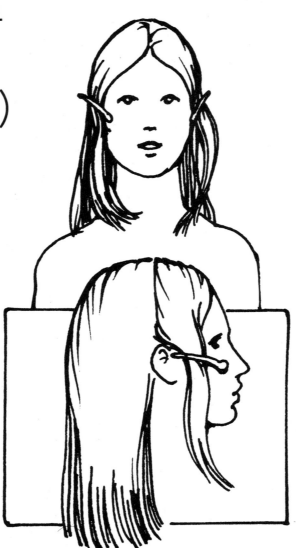
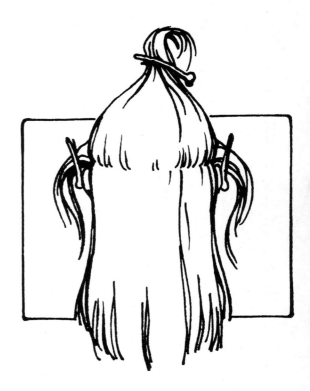

Step 1 Part wet clean hair from the hairline in the center of the crown. Then from the crown to just behind each ear (both left and right). Put these parted sections into a clip or rubber band (each side separately) and get it out of the way.

Step 2 With the remaining free hair, make a 1-inch parting from the bottom hairline up, from ear to ear, comb it down and put the rest up out of the way.

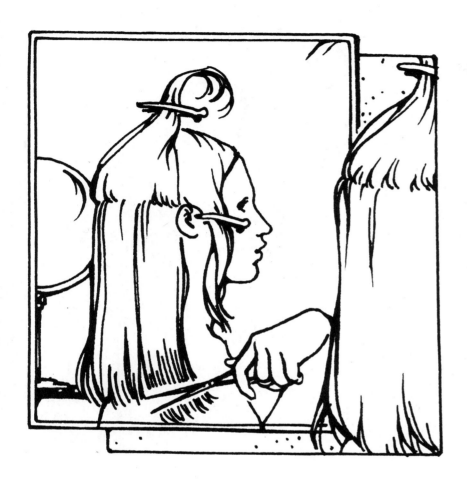 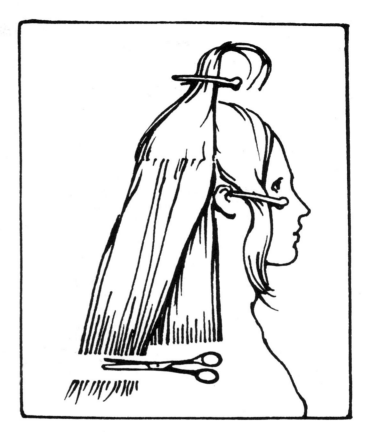

Step 3 Looking in two mirrors, comb the 1-inch parting down straight and cut off as much as you wish from ear to ear in an oval shape (or straight across if you wish).

Step 4 From the large section of hair you have pinned up in the back, go up another 1 inch with the comb and make another parting from ear to ear, following the line of the first parting. Bring this new hair down over what you have just cut, and tie up the rest again. Comb the new part down and using your first cut as a guide, cut the hair 1/4 inch longer than the first cut.

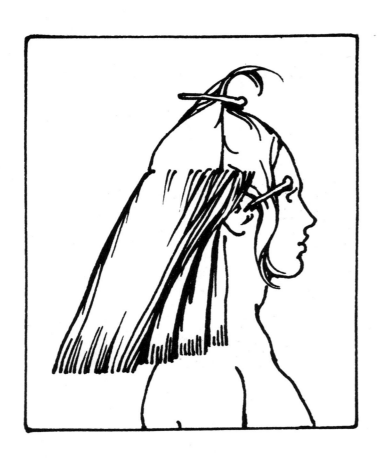

Step 5 Take another 1-inch parting, bring it down, and repeat Step 4—leaving a 1/4-inch overhang before you cut. Do this all the way up until you reach a point about 1 inch over the top of the ear.

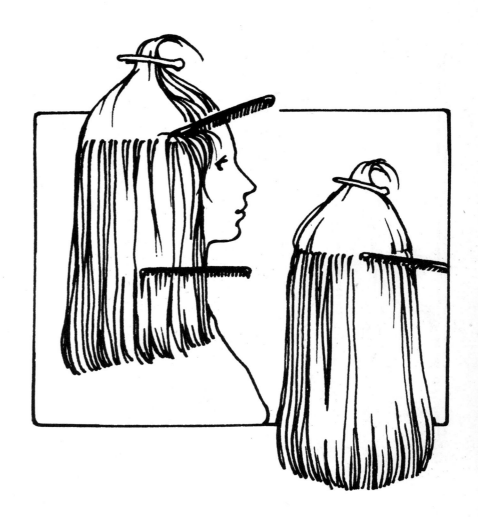

Step 6 Take down the right side of the hair you have pinned up. With the comb, make a part about 1 inch over the top of your ear. Go straight back to the center of the back of your head and comb straight down.

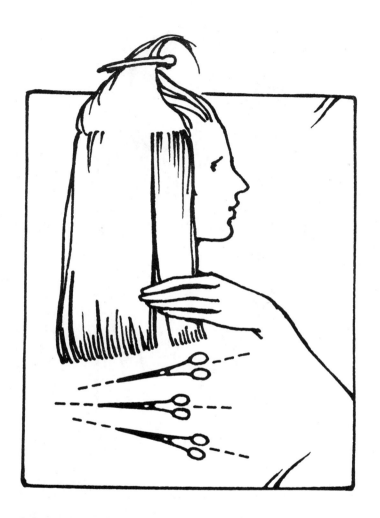

Step 7 Holding this new side part down, cut it to meet the back section, which has just been cut. This can be shorter or longer or the same length as the back depending on the style you want.

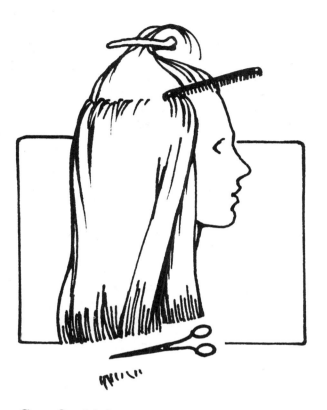

Step 8 Make a parting up another 1 inch—following the line you have just made from front to back. Bring down another section and cut it 1/4 inch longer than the last.

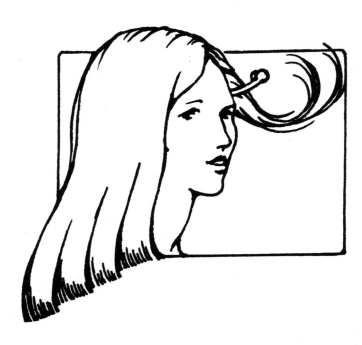

Step 9 Do this until all the hair on the side has been cut, section after section.

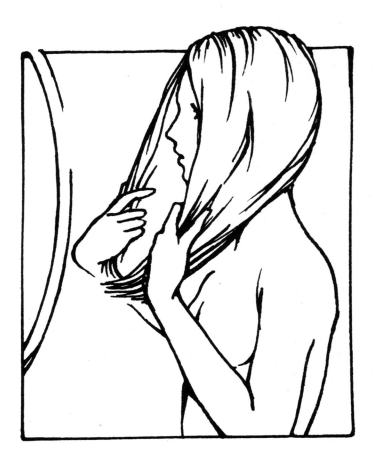

Step 10 Take down the left side and repeat what you have just done on the right, starting 1 inch over the top of the ear. If you cannot judge the first cut here, so that it is equal to the other side, simply pull the hair forward, measure it with the other side, and cut a little section to begin as a guide for the other side to be cut.

This haircut can be worn just as it is—or you can add bangs. Follow the next 7 steps to cut bangs.

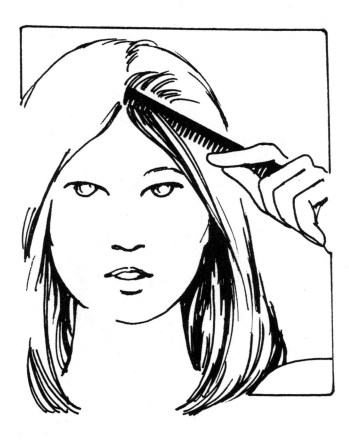

Step 11 With your hair parted in the middle, place your comb to make a parting about 1½ inch from your front hairline back along the middle part. Right side first.

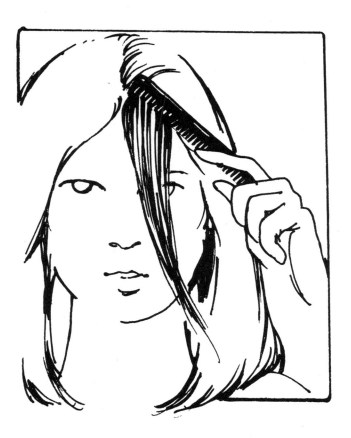

Step 12 Using the comb—make a line parting on an angle down toward the end of your right eyebrow.

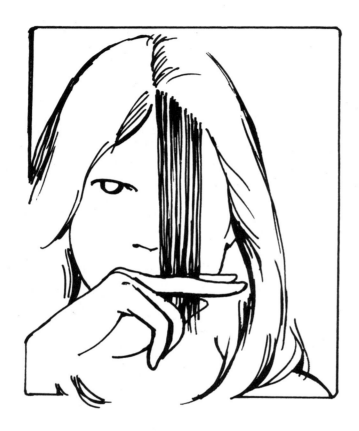

Step 13 Bring this triangular section forward and comb straight down over your face.

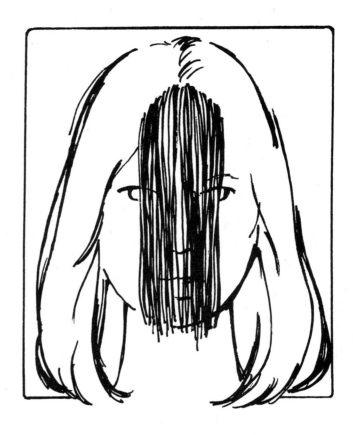

Step 14 Do the same on the left side.

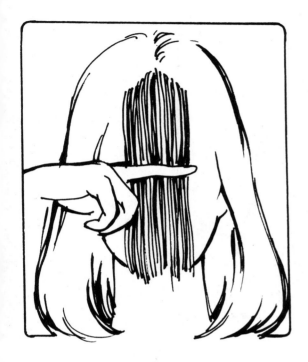 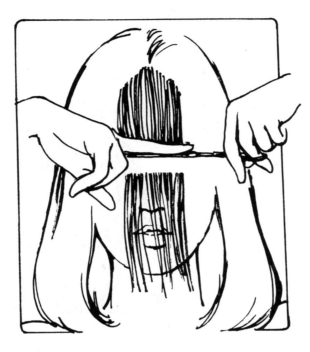 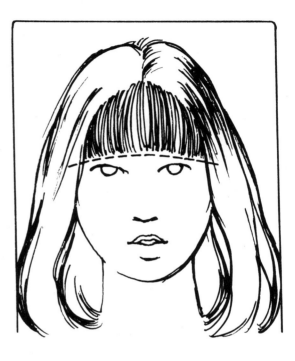

Step 15 Now, using the two fingers of the hand you do not cut with, comb and hold hair down. (You will have to look *through* your hair into the mirror—but this *is* possible.) Position your fingers at the indentation ridge on top of your nose.

Step 16 Put down the comb and pick up the scissors with your cutting hand. Cut just *below* your fingers.

Step 17 When you have finished and the bangs *dry*, they will be shorter. If they are still too long—*when dry*—trim edges, in a slight arc.

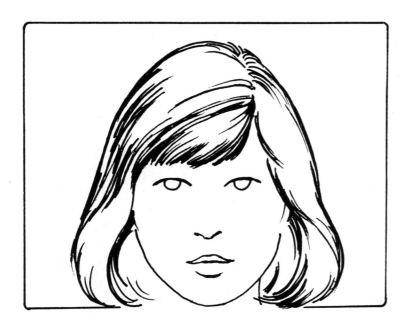

Parted on the side.

The completed haircut can be worn in different ways.

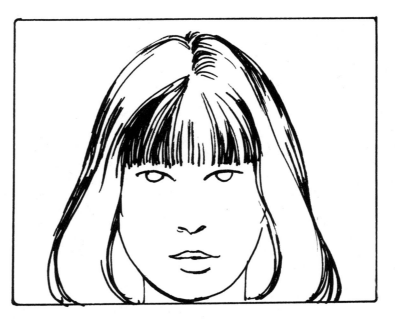

Straight across.

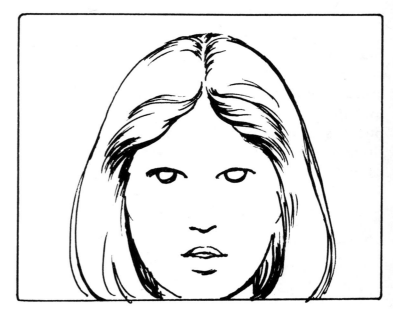

Bangs pushed back to the sides.

5 How to Cut Children's Hair

In this chapter we will show three haircuts, under two categories—Short and Long. You can use your own judgment as to whether or not the preceding chapters are more relevant to your child's hair. This chapter is really for very young children with fairly short hair, or with hair long enough to braid or tie back.

Note: The second example in this chapter (the child with the very curly hair) can be very useful also for men and women with very curly hair.

Short Hair —Straight

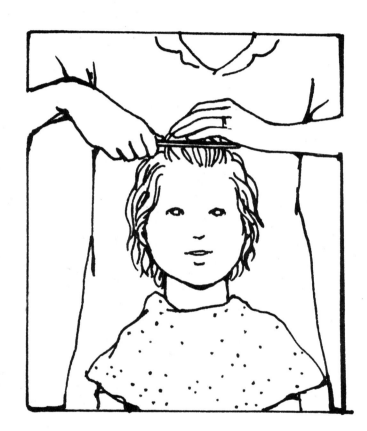

Step 1 Comb wet clean hair straight back away from the face.

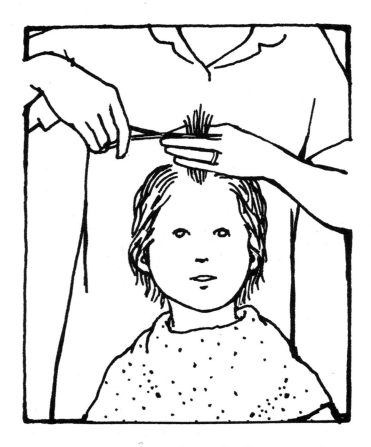

Step 2 Begin by combing the hair straight up at the center of the head and cutting off whatever you have decided upon.

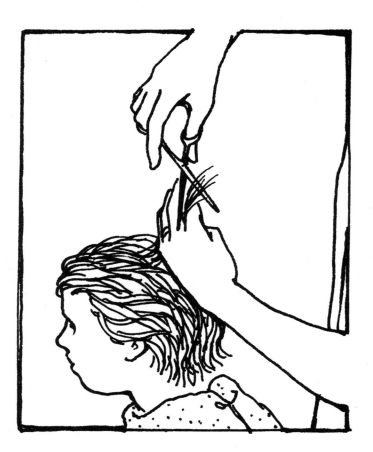

Step 3 Continue this process of combing up and cutting the hair all the same length until you reach the crown of the head.

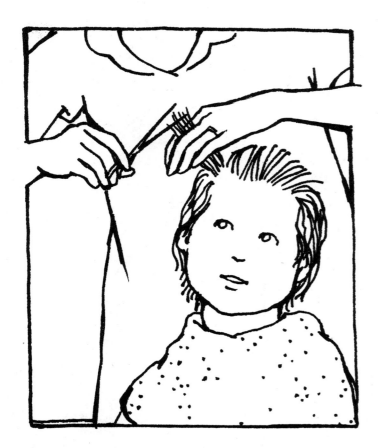

Step 4 Go back to the front and start on one side and do the same thing. Comb the hair straight out and cut it on an angle conforming to the shape of the head. Do this all the way to the center of the back of the head.

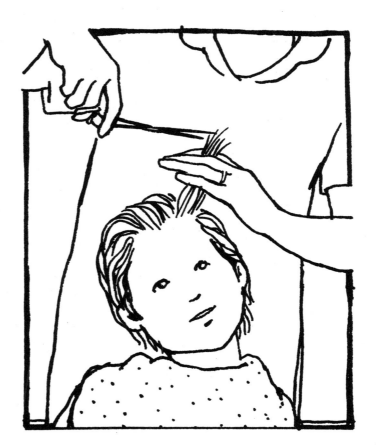

Step 5 Now do the other side the same way.

Step 6 When you have come this far you will have cut all but the very back part of the head the same length. Cut this section by starting on one side and working toward the other (left to right), and cut it the same length as you have the rest, using what you have already cut as a guide.

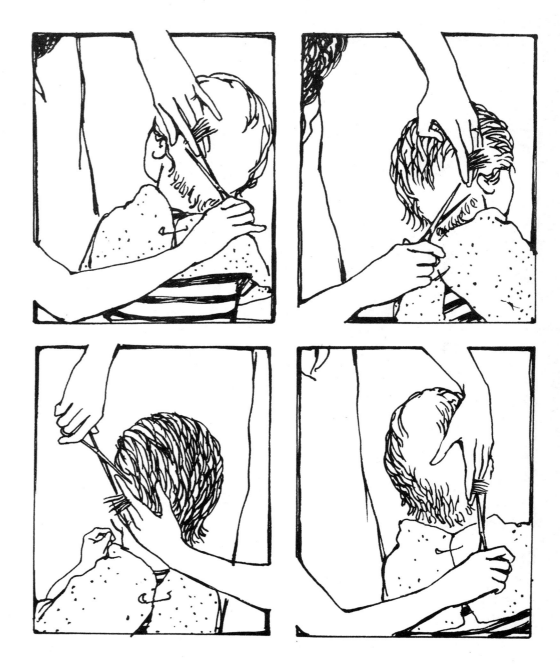

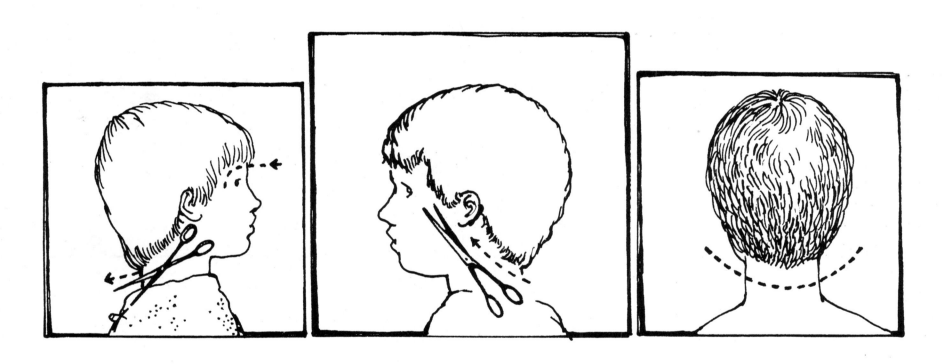

Step 7 Comb all the hair straight down from the crown of the head and cut off the edges all the way around—bangs included. You can make this last cutting as straight or as ragged as you wish.

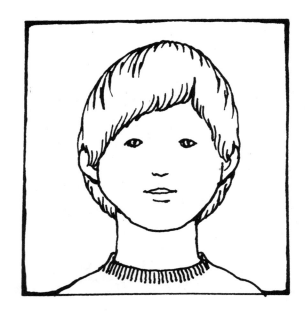 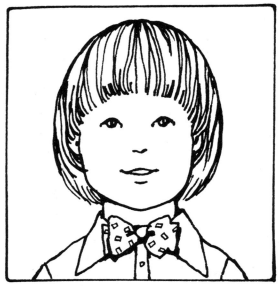 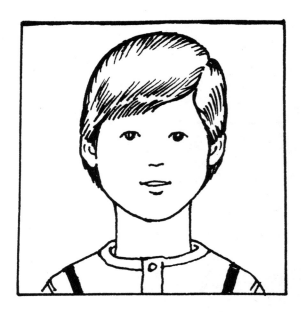

When you are finished it should look like this.

Short Hair —Curly

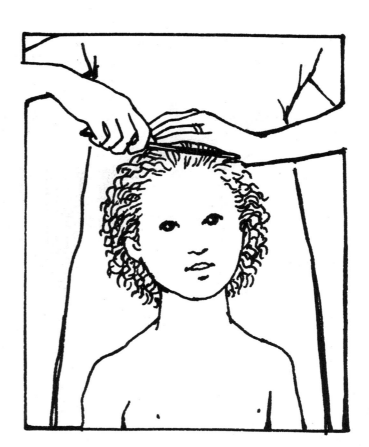

Step 1 Comb wet clean hair straight back away from the face.

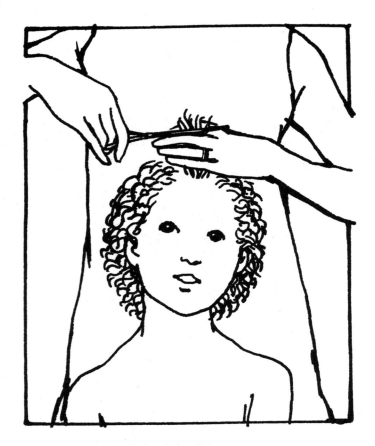

Step 2 Begin by combing the hair straight up at the center of the head and cutting off whatever you have decided upon.

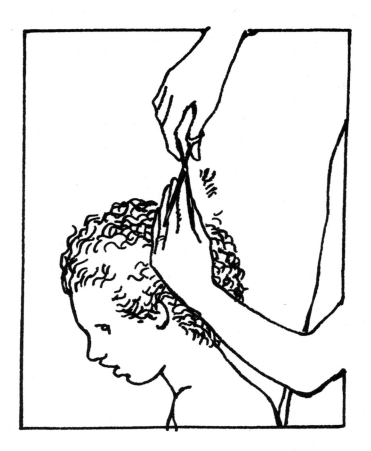

Step 3 Continue this process of combing up and cutting the hair all the same length until you reach the crown of the head.

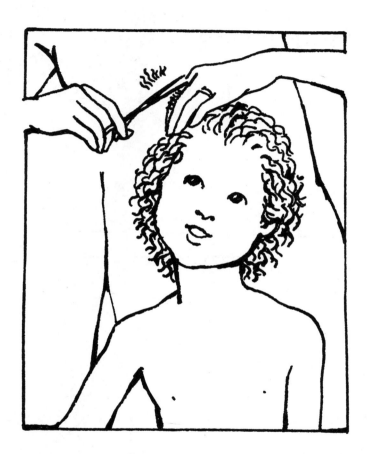

Step 4 Go back to the front and start on one side and do the same thing. Comb the hair straight out and cut it on an angle conforming to the shape of the head. Do this all the way to the center of the back of the head.

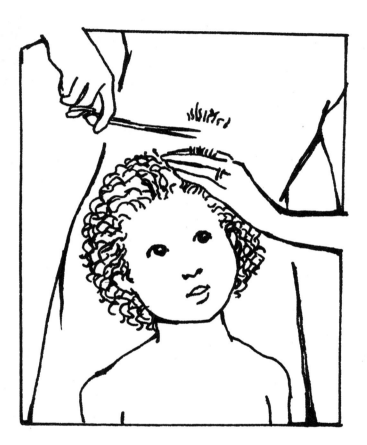

Step 5 Now do the other side the same way.

Step 6 When you have come this far you will have cut all but the very back part of the head the same length. Cut this section by starting on one side and working toward the other (left to right), and cut it the same length as you have the rest, using what you have already cut as a guide.

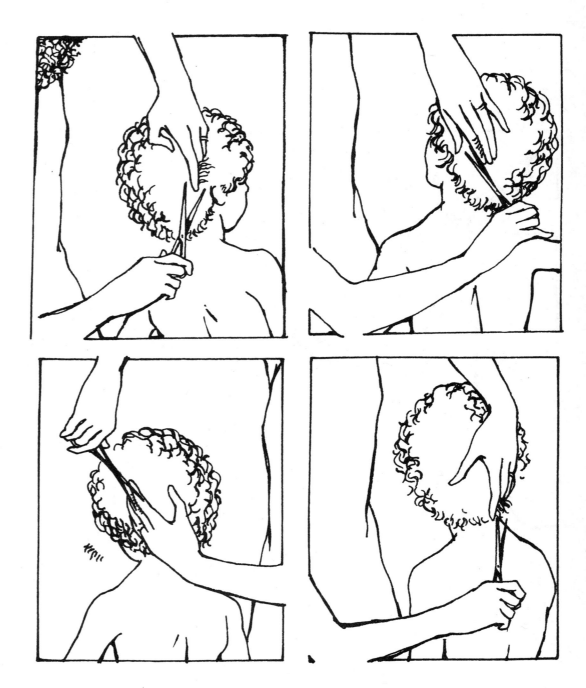

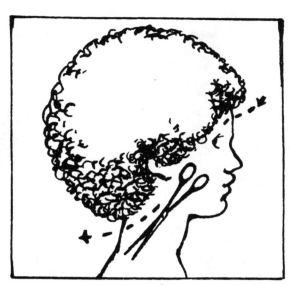 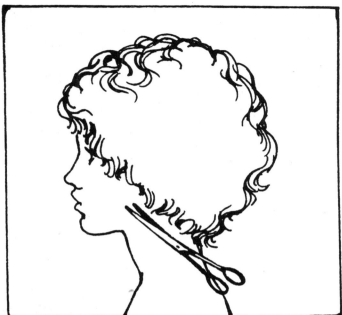 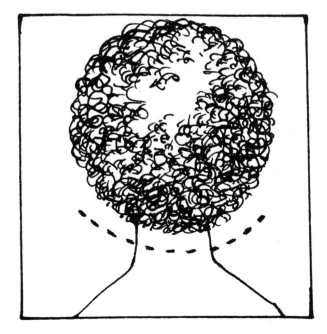

Step 7 Comb all the hair straight down from the crown of the head and cut off the edges all the way around—bangs included. You can make this last cutting as straight or as ragged as you wish.

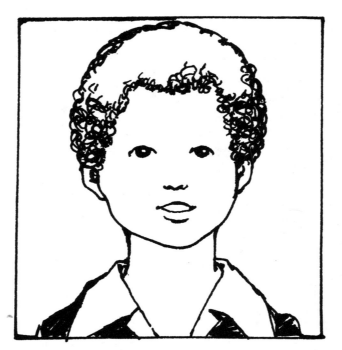
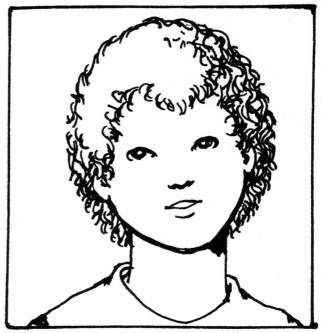

When you are finished it should look like this.

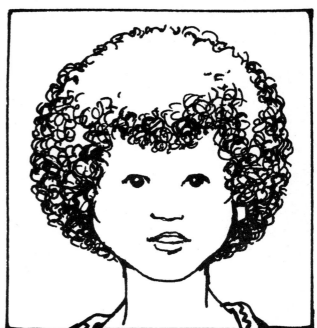

Long Hair

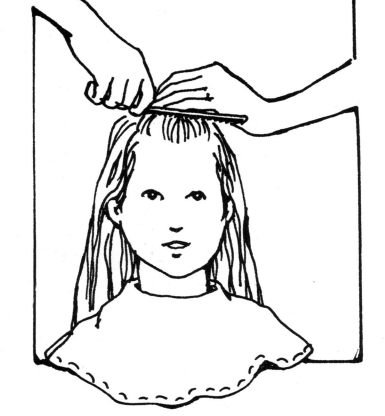

Step 1 Comb wet clean hair straight back away from the face.

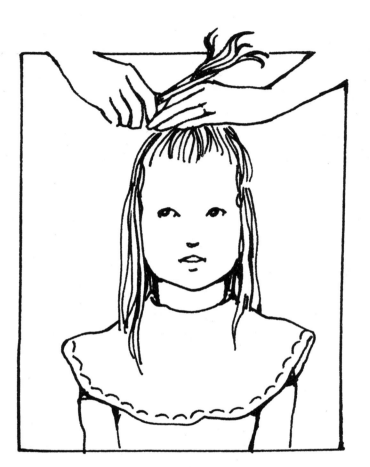 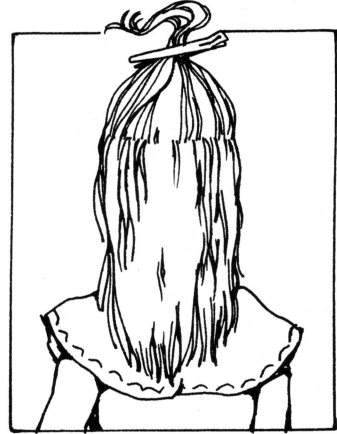

Step 2 With the comb, make a parting from above the ear on the left all the way around the head to the same spot above the right ear, and comb this hair down. Put up the rest of the hair in a clip to get it out of the way.

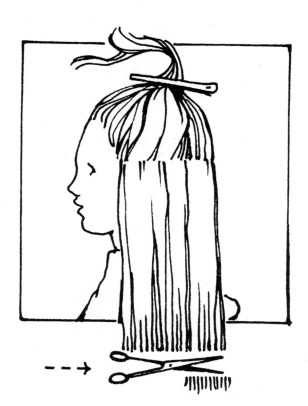 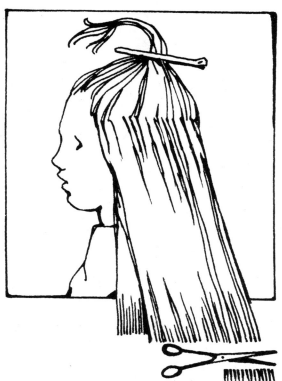 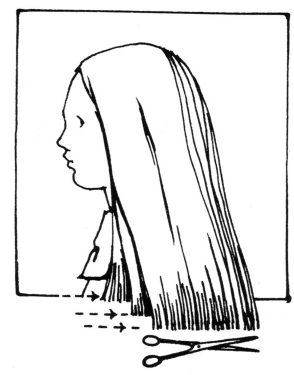

Step 3 Cut the hair all around as short as you wish, making it straight across or slightly angled toward the back.

Step 4 Bring down about half of the remaining hair, making the part exactly parallel to the first one you made...from the middle of the forehead on the left side to the same spot on the right. Comb the hair down and cut it 1/4 inch longer than you did on the first cut, following the cut hair closely as a guide.

Step 5 Bring down the rest of the hair and repeat. (Cut it 1/4 inch longer than your last cut.)

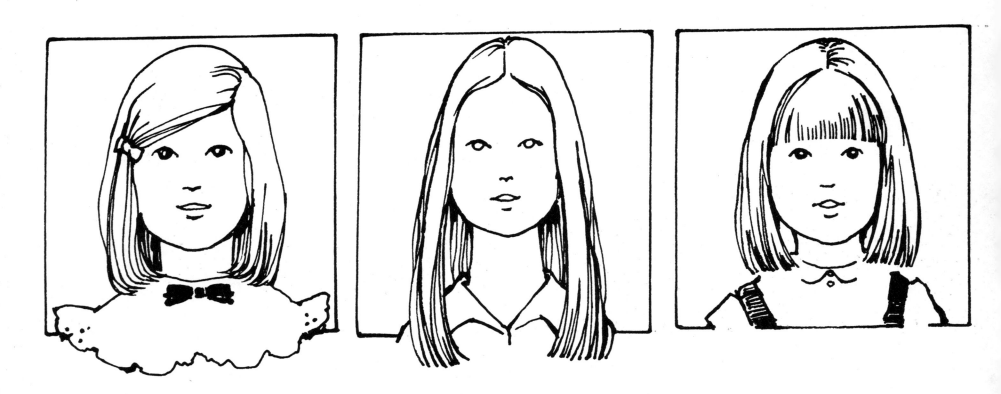

When you are finished it should look like this.

6
How to Blow-Dry Your Hair

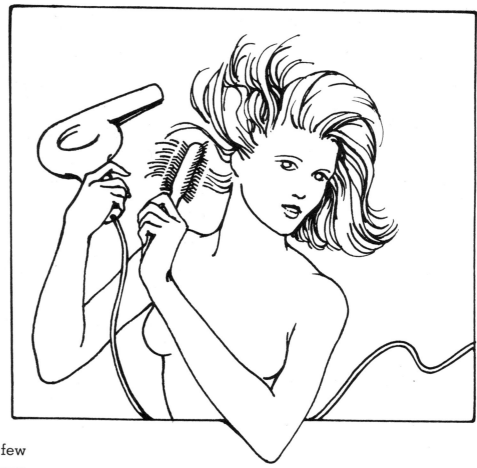

Before you begin to blow-dry your hair, let me offer a few hints. After shampooing and towel-drying your hair, use a large flat brush and move your hair around all over your head, using the blower to remove all the excess water. Brush and blow your hair in all directions until it it almost dry. This applies for both short and long hair. Then, comb your hair into the style you want, and follow the illustrations.

Long Hair Turned Under

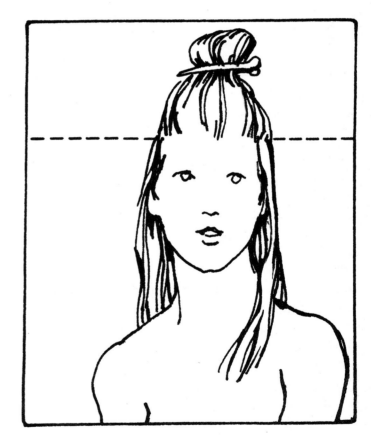

Step 1 Divide the hair in half, putting the top half in a clip.

Step 2 Using a circular brush, follow with the dryer to the ends and curl under.

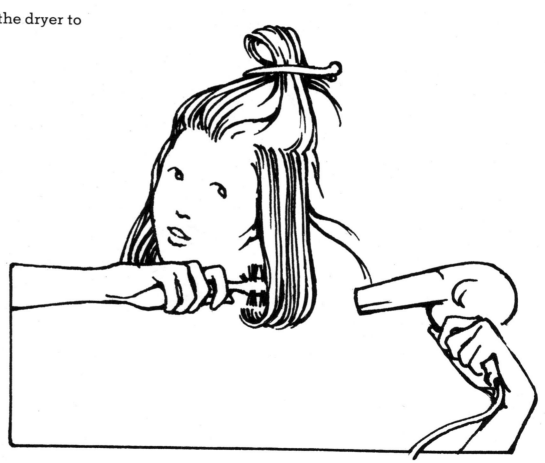

Step 3 Do this all the way around the head.

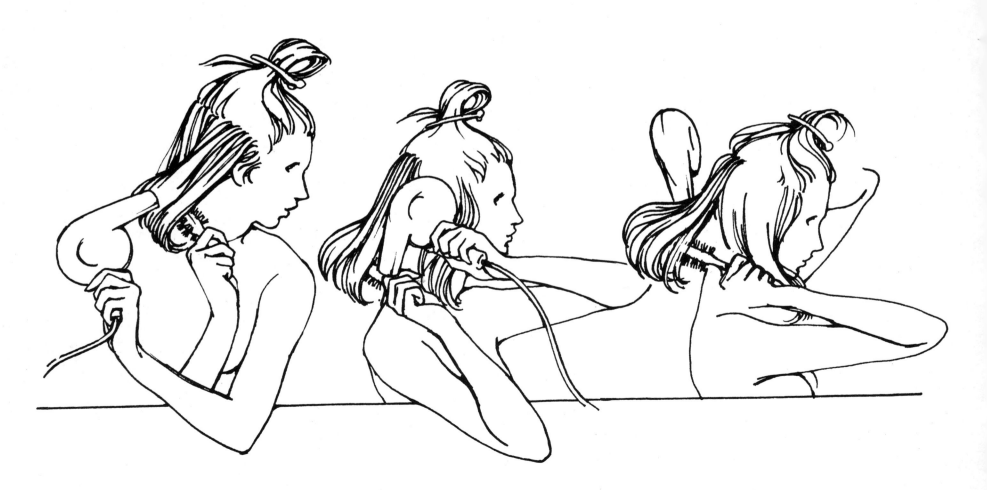

Step 4 Take down the top half and repeat, drying the hair slightly up from the scalp and turning under.

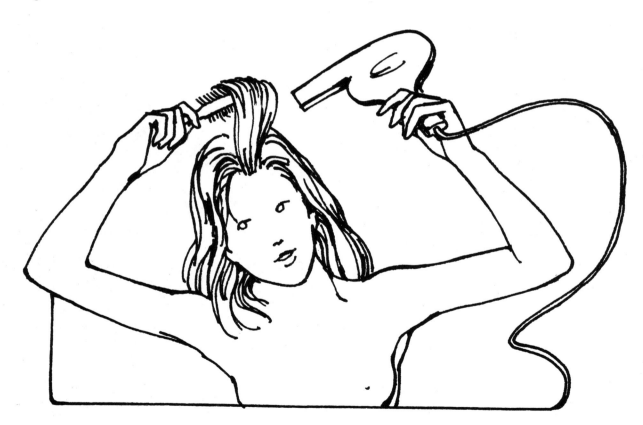

Step 5 Complete the top half all the way around and when finished...

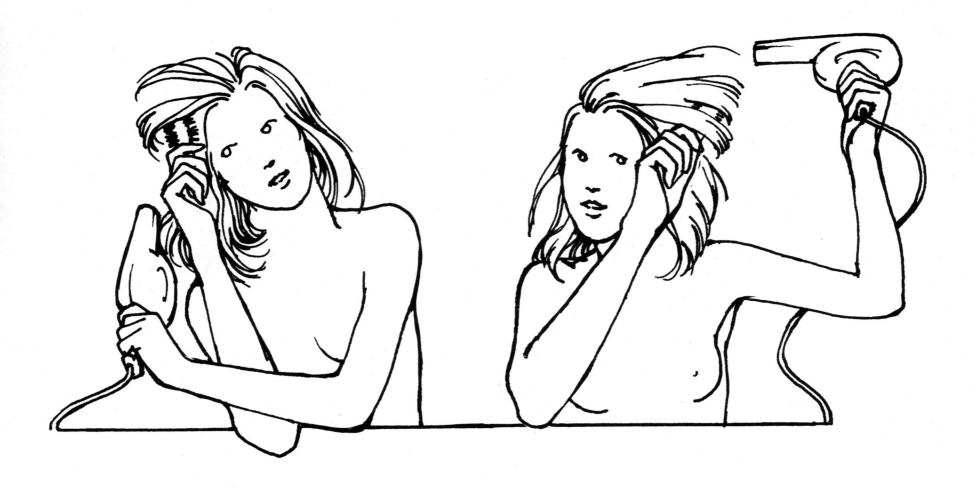

Step 6 brush under.

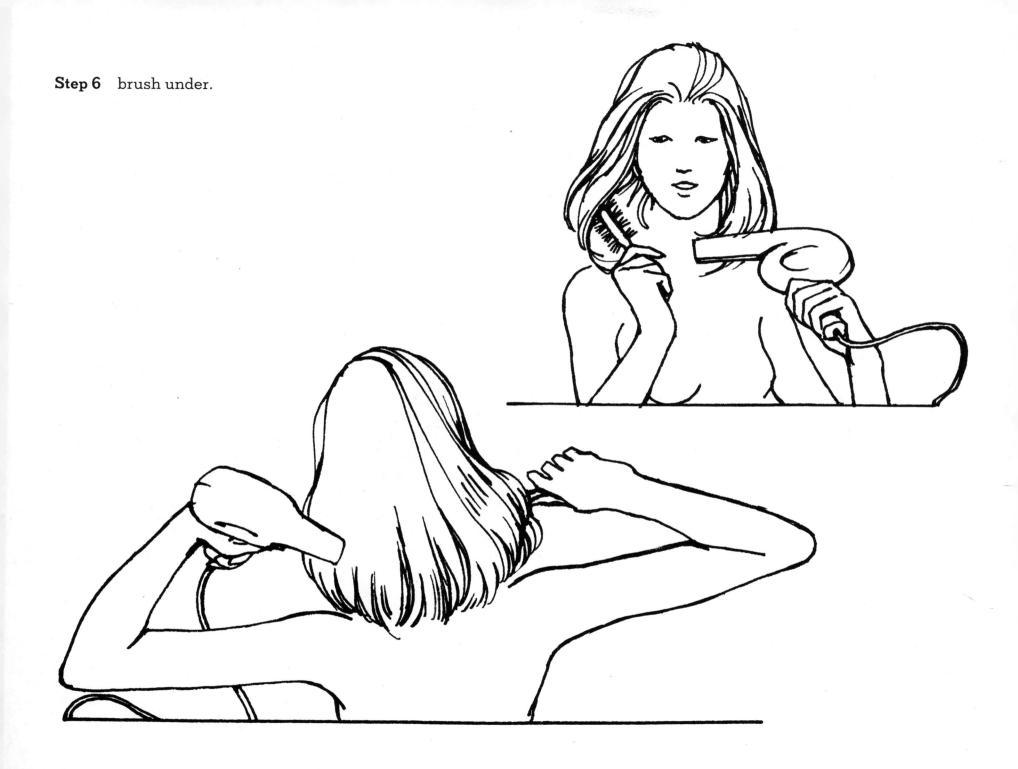

Long Hair Turned Up (Flip)

Follow the instructions and illustrations in previous style, but roll the hair around the brush in the opposite direction (pointing up).

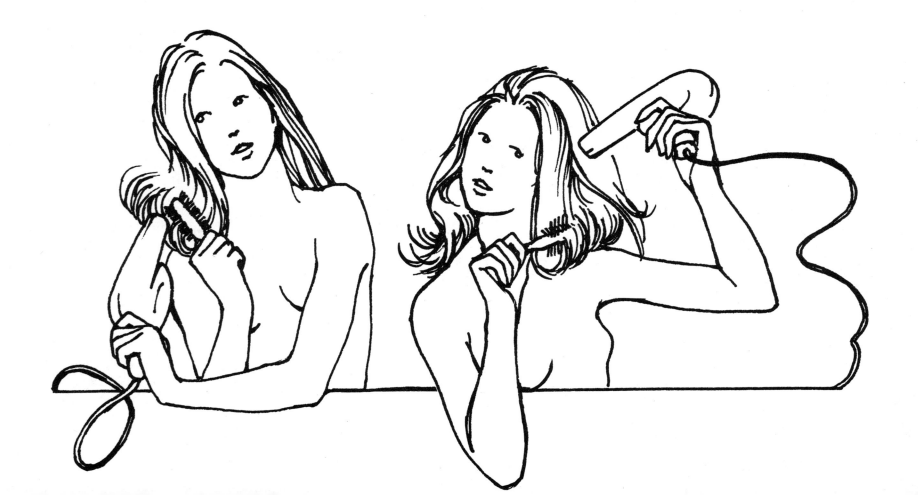

Short Hair Away from the Face

Step 1 With a circular brush (as small as you can find), start at the front hairline and make small partings, curling the hair around the brush and directing the warm air toward the brush with the dryer.

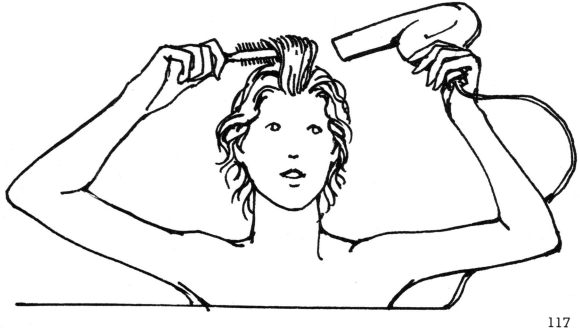

Step 2/ Go back about an inch and repeat to the crown.

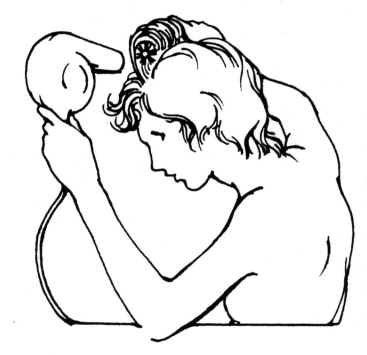

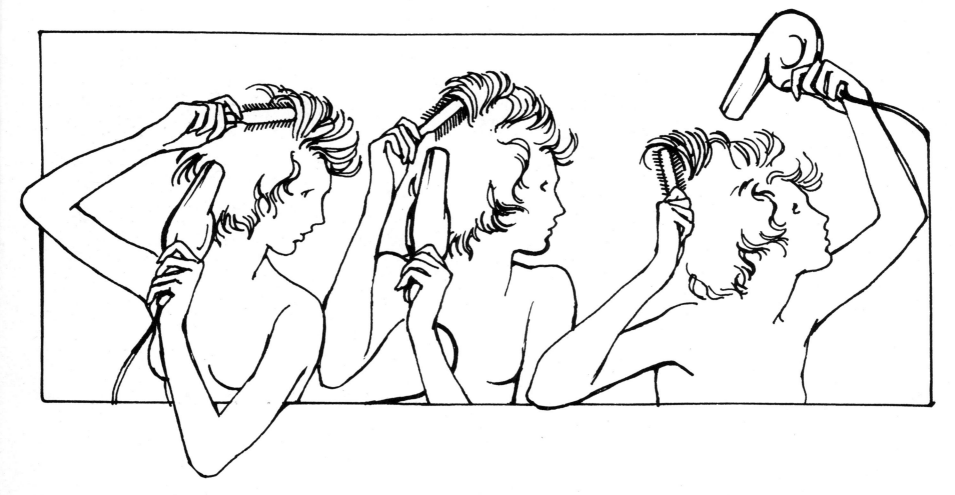

Step 3 Do the same on each side.

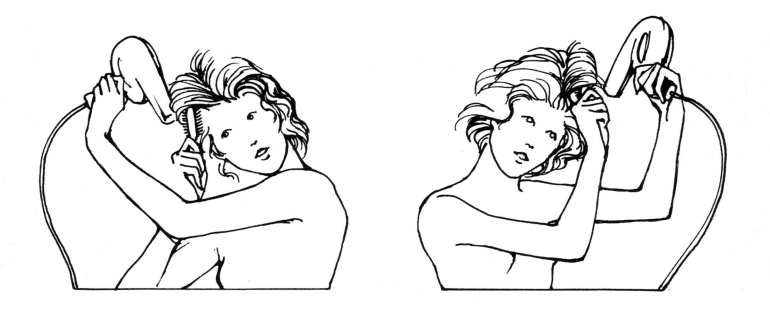

Step 4 The very back and bottom of the head can be done by first curling the hair around the brush with both hands, and then directing the air at what you have turned around the brush. Turn everything under and when you are finished—comb the hair any way you want. The important thing is to dry it with a slight curl.

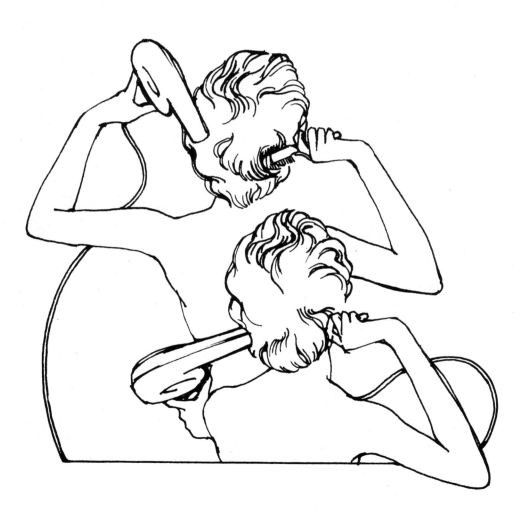

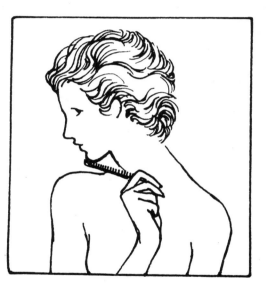

Short Hair Toward the Face

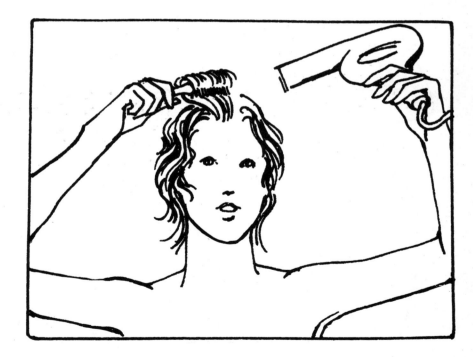

Step 1 Start at the crown and curl some hair around the brush and dry.

Step 2 Take another inch or so of hair in front of that and repeat.

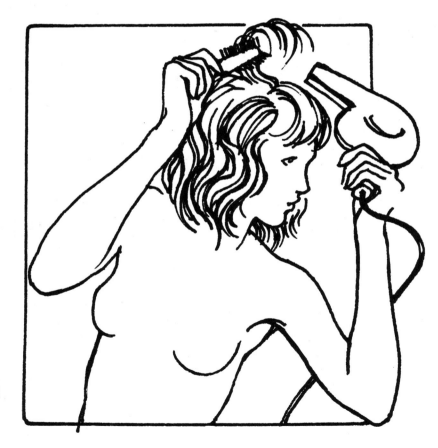

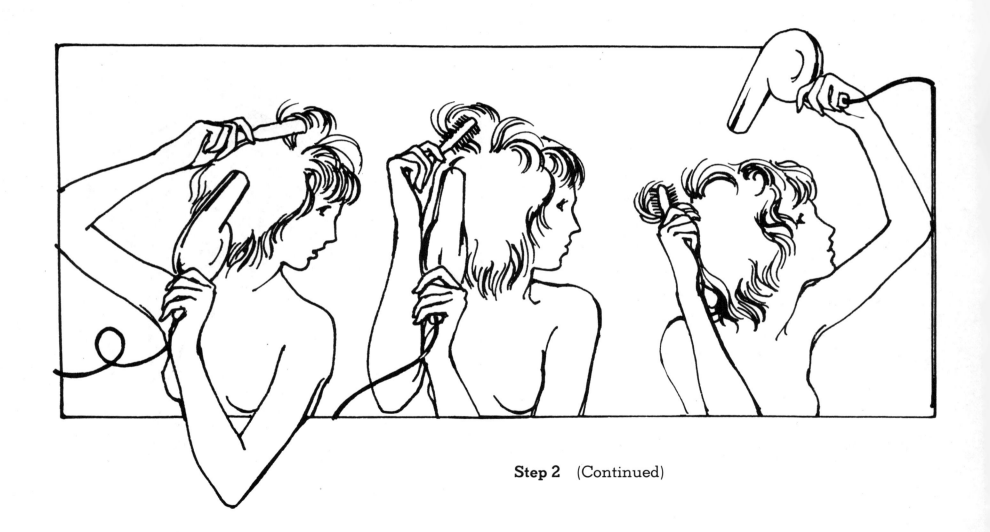

Step 2 (Continued)

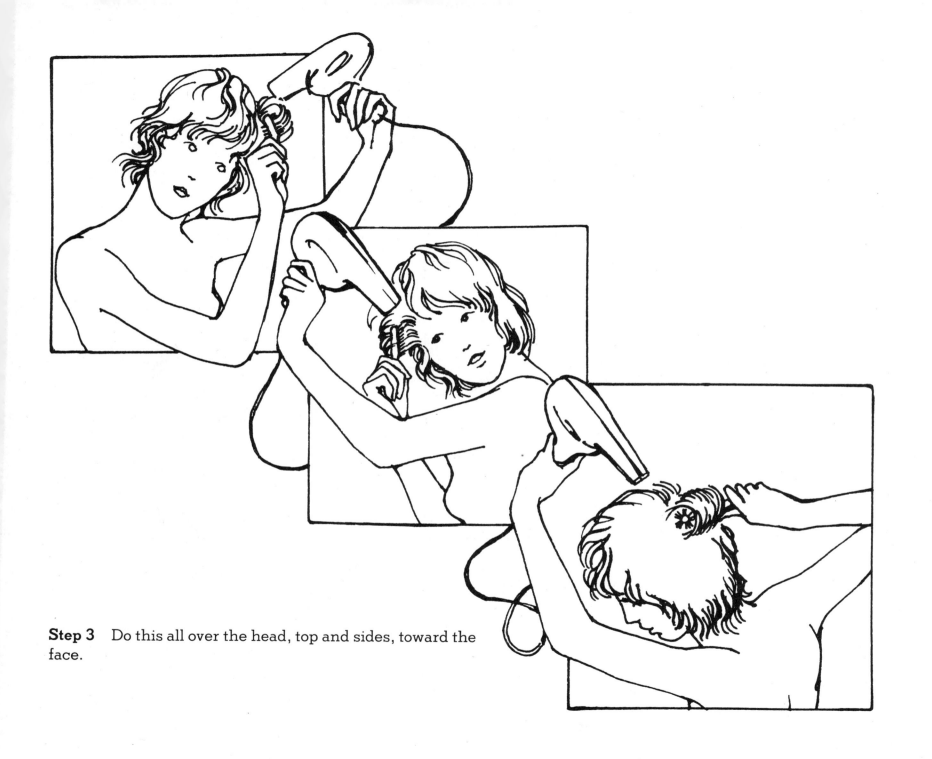

Step 3 Do this all over the head, top and sides, toward the face.

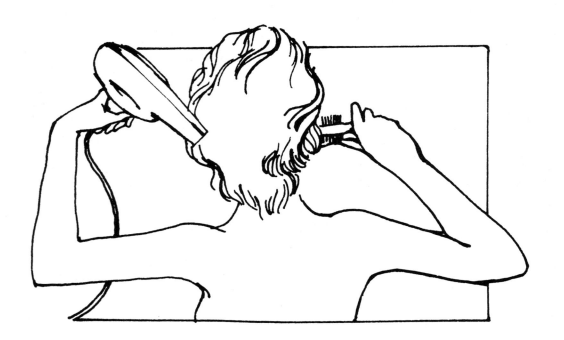 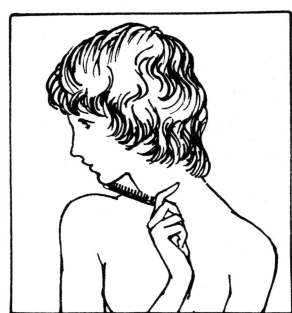

Step 4 Curl the back and the bottom as before (blow-dry 3) and comb as you wish.

Men's Hair

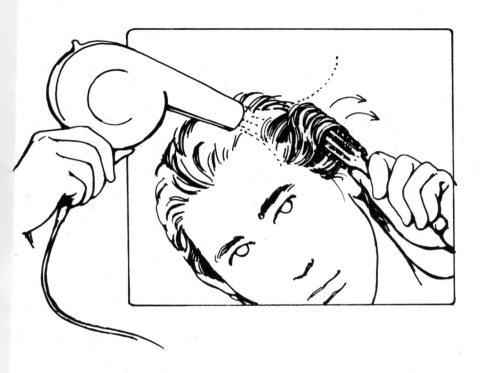

Step 1 Blow all the layers rolling the hair slightly *under* with a round brush.

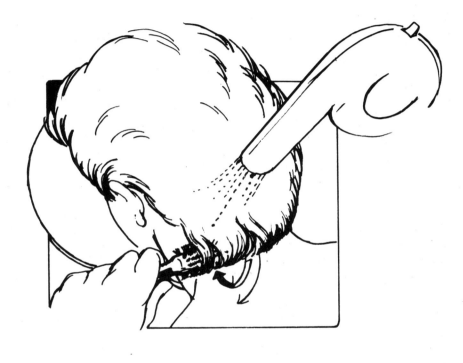

Step 2 Do this all over the head especially at the back of the head around the nape of the neck. Roll *under*.

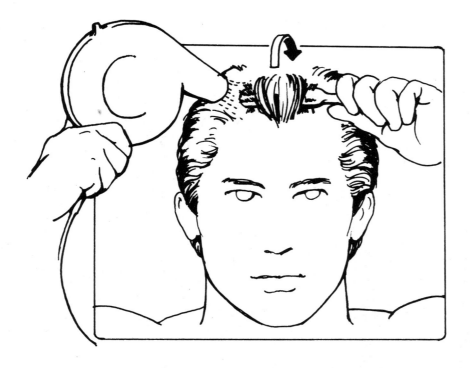

Step 3 Finish by blowing the top and front of your hair back.

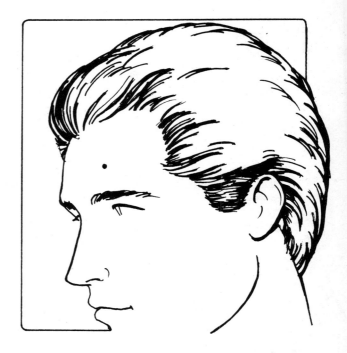

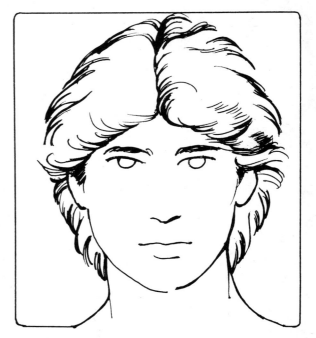